ANATOMY OF
A BUILDING

First published in Great Britain in 2014 by Little, Brown

Copyright © Royal College of Physician 2014

The moral right of the author has been asserted.

Picture credits: p 9 © Geremy Butler; p 10, 12, 13, 25, 26, 30, 31, 32 (bottom), 34, 38 (bottom), 41 (all), 42, 44/45, 51, 53, 71, 76, 77, 78, 79 (top), 81, 82, 85, 86, 92, 94, 95, 99, 105, 110, 112 © Hélène Binet; p 15 (top) © Architectural Press Archive/RIBA Library Photographs Collection; p 15 (bottom), 38 (top) © RIBA Library Photographs Collection; p 16/17 © Lasdun Archive/RIBA Library Photographs Collection; page 18, 56, 59, 61, 91 © Getty Images; p 19 © Richard Bryant/Arcaid; p 23 © Henk Snoek / RIBA Library Photographs Collection; p 24, 27, 97 © John Donat/RIBA Library Photographs Collection; p 28, 29, 48, 106 © Mike Fear/Royal College of Physicians; p 28 (right hand image), 47 © The Edge; p 32 (top), 84 © Niall Clutton; p 37 (all), 63 © UIG via Getty Images; p 40, 54/55, 58, 67, 68, 69, 70, 75 (top), 80, 102, 103 © Royal College of Physicians; p 60 © National Portrait Gallery, London; p 64 © View Pictures/Rex; p 73, 79 (bottom), 93, 96, 98, 100, 108/109 © HUFTON + CROW; p 75 (bottom) © Niall Clutton/Royal College of Physicians; p 87 © Mark David Hill/Royal College of Physicians; p 88 © James Partridge/Royal College of Physicians; p 89 © Mondadori via Getty Image.

Designed by Emil Dacanay and Sian Rance, D.R. ink

A CIP catalogue record for this book is available from the British Library.

ISBN 978-1-4087-0622-0

Printed and bound in Italy

500
REFLECTIONS
ON THE RCP
1518–2018

ANATOMY OF
A BUILDING
Rowan Moore

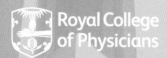
Royal College
of Physicians

FOREWORD

The Royal College of Physicians was founded, by Royal Charter, in 1518 by King Henry VIII. Few professional organisations have been in continuous existence for so long, and over its five-hundred-year history the College has been at the centre of many aspects of medical life. Its purpose is to promote the highest standards of medical practice in order to improve health and health care, and its varied work in the field is held in very high regard. Currently, the College has over thirty thousand members and fellows worldwide. Over the years it has accumulated a distinguished library, extensive archives, museum collections of portraits and other treasures, and has been housed in a number of notable buildings. As part of its quincentennial commemoration, a series of ten books has been commissioned, of which this is the first part. Each book features fifty items, thereby making a total of five hundred, and the series is intended to be a meditation on, and an exploration of, aspects of the College's work and collections over its five-hundred-year history.

This volume on the College buildings, written by the distinguished architectural writer and critic Rowan Moore, begins the series. It is a brilliant exposition of the structure, history and meaning of the College's buildings, with superb photography by Hélène Binet and Nick Hufton, among others – this a memorable book to launch the collection.

Grateful thanks are due to many persons who have contributed to the series. First, to Professor Linda Luxon, Treasurer of the College, who has had the vision to promote and oversee the project. I would like also to express the College's gratitude to Orla Fee, Tom Grinyer and Julie Beckwith, and others in its Communications Department, who have worked tirelessly and provided enormous assistance in the preparation of the books. Finally, also, I thank Adam Strange at Little, Brown, the publisher, and Sian Rance, the book designer, for their expert work on behalf of the College.

Simon Shorvon

Simon Shorvon, Harveian Librarian, Royal College of Physicians Series Editor

CONTENTS

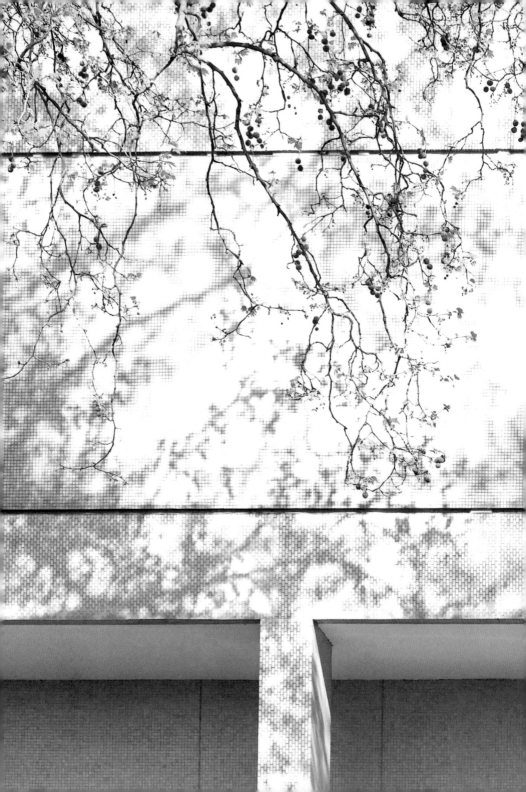

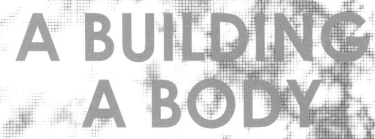

A BUILDING, A BODY

'a space that oscillates between
reason and feeling'

BODY AND BUILDING

The most persistent idea in Western architecture is that there are affinities between the human figure and buildings. It is present in everyday language – a building can have a heart, skin, face (façade), guts, legs – and Michelangelo compared columns and pilasters to bones and sinews. It is present in the ancient idea that the classical orders corresponded with human types: Doric was a man, Ionic a woman, Corinthian a girl. The role of symmetry in architecture, usually about one axis, can be related to that of the face and body. Bodies and buildings both need circulation.

The concept can be expanded to place humans and buildings in a chain of resemblances that includes cities and the universe. 'A house is a small city,' said the Renaissance theorist and architect Leon Battista Alberti. In Mycenaean palaces can be found large circular hearths, *omphaloi*, which were conceived as the centre of the building, as the navel or midpoint of the human body, as the point of connection between this world and others, and as the ideal centre of the cosmos. One of the most famous drawings in history is Leonardo's Vitruvian Man, in which a naked figure is inscribed within a circle centred on his navel, and a square. Its purpose is to demonstrate the proportions believed to govern both the body and the universe, as Leonardo's notes make clear, which could also be applied to architecture.

> **The most persistent idea in Western architecture is that there are affinities between the human figure and buildings – a building can have a heart, skin, face guts, and legs**

In the seventeenth-century anatomical theatre in the University of Bologna, tiers rise around a central slab on which a body would be dissected. In the ceiling, directly above the cadaver, are symbolic representations of Zodiacal constellations. It is an explicit re-statement of the analogy of body and universe, in which architectural space was an intermediate term.

But, in the same time and place that this symbolism was affirmed, it was undermined by the activities of what the theatre contained. Scientific enquiry not only did violence to the bodies cut up for research, but it also dismembered the idea of the likeness of microcosm and macrocosm. In the Scientific Revolution, in parallel with the discoveries of the anatomists, astronomers like Kepler discovered that the universe is nothing like the centred, man-like, geometrically regular and finite thing implied by Leonardo's drawing.

Among the many consequences (and not the most significant of them) would be the slow unravelling of the certainties underlying classical architecture which, to cut a long story extremely short, would eventually contribute to the twentieth-century view that a new kind of architecture had to be found. Mostly this view did not entail a rejection or forgetting of the classical but a worrying-over it that could border on the obsessive. The aim was to recover and reinterpret what still had meaning from the past, and combine it with the forms of an age which was by now industrial.

The most influential examples of this thinking were the works and words of the Swiss-French architect Le Corbusier. In his book, *Vers Une Architecture* of 1923, he printed on facing pages images of the Parthenon and of what were then up-to-date and stylish cars. The juxtapositions were provocative, but also showed a desire to combine the classical and the mechanical. The same desire can be seen in Le Corbusier's buildings, which fused elements derived from temples and aeroplanes, and would use symmetries, proportions, columns and beams in ways which were still abstractly classical, but in unprecedented combinations.

An aspect of this architecture was a conception of space allied to that of Cubist art. As painters would break up the face or body into a series of overlapping planes, architects dissolved the boundaries of rooms and buildings, using glass walls and other devices, such that interior and exterior could interpenetrate. The body was still there – l e Corbusier would produce his own version of the Vitruvian Man, Le Modulor – but its integrity was put in question and its order rearranged. It was no longer possible to believe in the easy harmony of great and small. If wholeness was still desired, its achievement would be more complicated.

On display in the Royal College Physicians' headquarters are artefacts from the same century and country as the theatre in Bologna that represent a similar ambivalent urge to understand the body by taking it apart. These are the anatomical tables, pinewood boards on which the circulatory and nervous systems of executed criminals, having first been treated with a

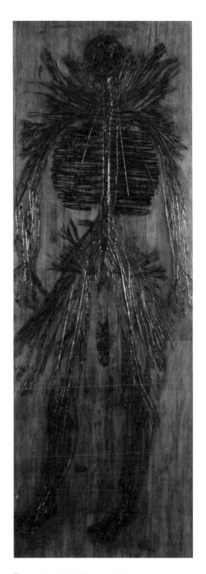

The anatomical tables are 'gruesome, skilful and exquisite'

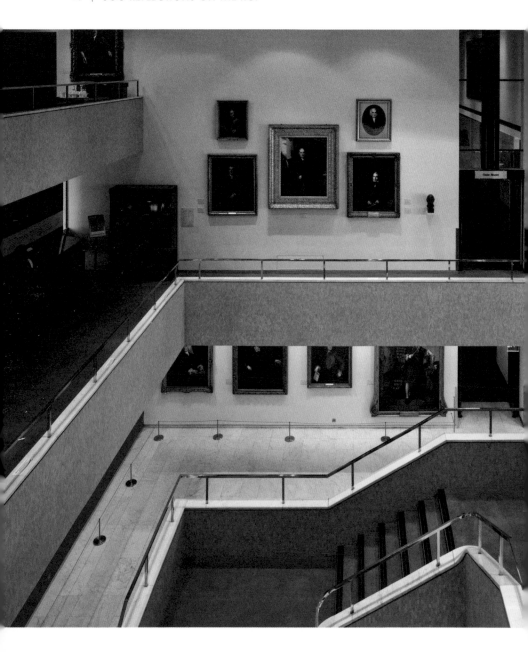

This triple-height hall can be called the heart of the College, its physical and symbolic centre

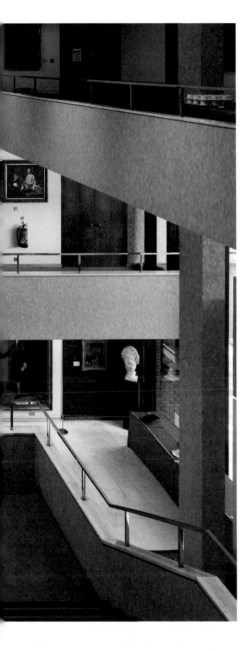

hardening agent and removed from their bodies, are laid out. They are gruesome, skilful and exquisite. The poses of these residual humans are arranged with a degree of art that indicates a concern for their former form, at the same time that that form has been meticulously destroyed in the pursuit of knowledge.

They hang alongside some of the College's ancestral portraits on the wall of a gallery that overlooks its Marble Hall. This triple-height hall, renamed the Lasdun Hall in 2014 in honour of its architect, can be called the heart of the College, its physical and symbolic centre, but in the place where a Mycenaean palace would have given you a hearth, a point of stability, here you find a poised and generous staircase. You get to the middle only to be invited to move somewhere else. The wish to make a centre is classical, but the restlessness, the centrifugal force, is modern.

From their boards the sightless nervous and circulatory systems contemplate a fine example of post-Cubist architectural space. (To be more precise the architect of the building, Denys Lasdun, credited the influence of Paul Klee, who was not Cubist, but who had a related spatial sensibility.) One face of the Marble Hall's cuboid volume is omitted, opening the space to a garden beyond. The view, however, is not uninterrupted, but punctuated by a smaller cuboid here seen from outside of itself, which contains the Censors' Room. Beyond the garden a degree of enclosure is achieved by the stucco façades of the John Nash buildings that pre-existed Lasdun's work, and by the long low hump in blue brick, part of the Lasdun construction, that

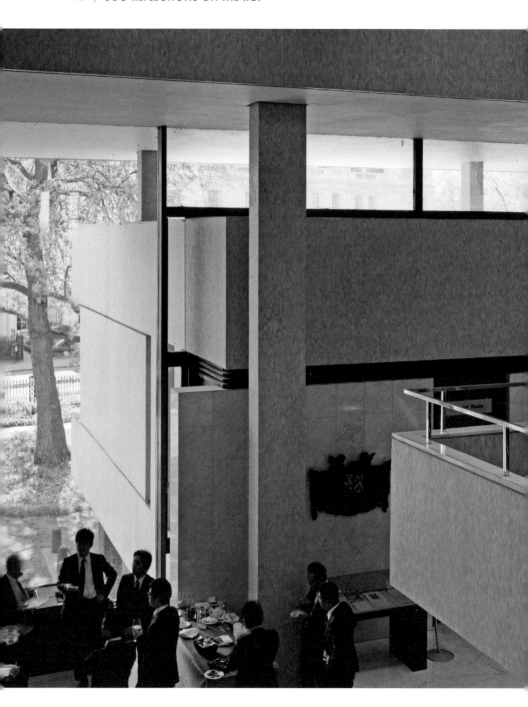

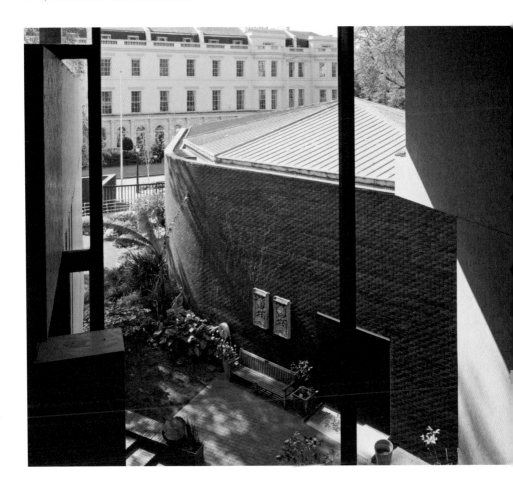

contains the College's Wolfson Theatre. This enclosure is incomplete and provisional: space continues to open up beyond it, into the rest of the city, the sky and infinity. It is a three-dimensional collage that cannot be considered or known from a single fixed point but through the accumulation of experiences over time.

The most important spatial distinction in a building, as in a body, is usually between outside and inside, and what passes from one to the other by whatever route is a matter of some concern, but here this distinction is sometimes made to disappear. A flow of space is aimed at, ultimately unlimited, but modulated and layered by the large box which you occupy, the small box that you contemplate, the garden, theatre and Nash façades. Detail and material reinforce the effect – the mosaic used to clad the exterior runs inside and outdoor materials like marble and brick are used within. The framing of the glass is often made to disappear so as not to disrupt the illusion.

DENYS LASDUN

The architect of the Royal College of Physicians' building in Regents Park, Denys Lasdun, was forty-four years old at the time that he was commissioned in 1958. Lasdun was one of the foremost British exponents of Corbusian architecture, but this description does not do justice to the way he forged his own powerful artistic personality.

As a student at the Architectural Association in London, he was profoundly impressed by *Vers Une Architecture* and stuck to its principles for his sixty-year career, even as he interpreted and enlarged them. On a visit to Paris he was bowled over by Le Corbusier's Pavillon Suisse, a building for students in the Cité Universitaire. He became 'very excited', as he later put it, by 'a substance; a muddy mixture of marl, clay, lime, sand, gravel, water, heavily laced with steel – reinforced concrete'. Finding his place of education obsessed with arcane debates as to which kind of Chinese ink to use, he 'could not get out of the AA fast enough'. He spent long enough there, however, to learn from its traditional classical education something about the principles of organising and planning buildings, derived from the École des Beaux Arts in Paris.

He went first to work for Wells Coates, whose Isokon apartment block in Lawn Road, Hampstead, was a confident early example of British modernism, the home for a while of Agatha Christie, as well as a refuge and stopping-off point for Walter Gropius, Marcel Breuer and other avant-garde escapees from Nazi Germany. According to William Curtis, author of a major book on Lasdun, Coates was 'a temporary artistic mentor' who taught the young architect 'the logic of a clear plan and the constructional details on which modern architecture relied'. Coates also imparted his belief, based on his knowledge of Japanese domestic design, in 'forms which serve life'.

In 1937 Lasdun designed, independently of Coates, a house in Newton Road, Paddington, whose pronounced horizontal windows show the clear influence of Le Corbusier's Maison Cook in Boulogne-sur-Seine. Later the home of Ronald Searle, creator of St Trinians, it was an extraordinarily confident building for a twenty-three year old and it still stands in striking contrast to its Victorian neighbours.

He next worked for Berthold Lubetkin who in the 1930s was the foremost exponent of the modern movement in Britain. His practice, called Tecton, designed the elliptical Penguin Pool at London Zoo, on whose intersecting spiral ramps the birds would until recently disport, as the architect had intended. Lubetkin also designed Highpoint I and II, apartment blocks in Highgate, described as 'the world's first vertical garden city', which jointly form one of the most successful examples anywhere of Le Corbusier's idea that high-rise living should be enriched by landscaping and sports facilities at ground level.

In the war Lasdun served with the Royal Artillery and then the Royal Engineers, landing on the continent shortly after D-Day, and helping to construct airstrips during the subsequent advance. With the peace he returned to Tecton, became a partner, and worked on the Hallfield housing estate in Paddington, a short distance from the Newton Road house. In 1948 Tecton dissolved, but Lasdun continued to work with Lindsay Drake, a colleague from the practice. Later he teamed up with the leading modernists Maxwell Fry and Jane Drew to form Fry Drew Drake and Lasdun, which lasted until 1959, although this was essentially a business arrangement: it was written into their contract that they would not design together, and Lasdun by now had his own separate architectural identity. Lubetkin, as the half-true legend has it, became disgusted with the practice of architecture and withdrew to farm pigs in Gloucestershire.

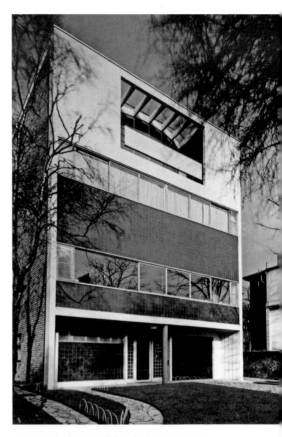

Lasdun started his post-Tecton career confidently, with Hallfield School, on the Hallfield Estate. It is a series of pavilions interspersed with sheltered outdoor spaces, connected to a sinuous central block in a way that Lasdun compared to petals on a stalk. It remains one of Lasdun's most successful buildings: it has clear echoes of Lubetkin, but has a freedom and inventiveness that are Lasdun's own. His use of quasi-organic forms, at a time when the rectangular grid was dominant in architecture, foreshadows a future interest in thinking of buildings as landscapes, as man-made versions of natural phenomena.

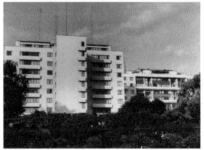

TOP: 32 Newton Road, Paddington, London
BOTTOM: Highpoint I and II, Highgate, London

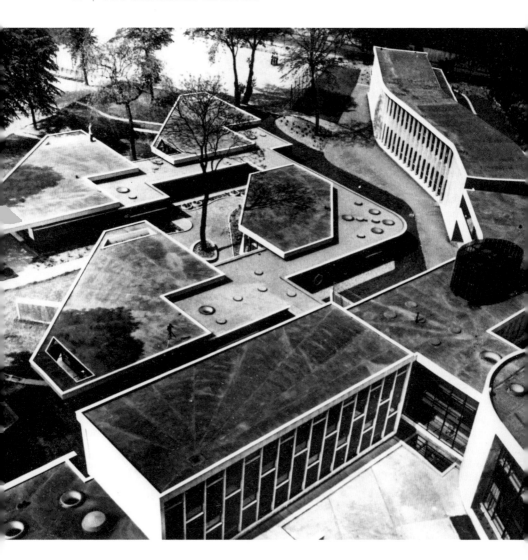

Lasdun's use of quasi-organic forms, at a time when the rectangular grid was dominant in architecture, foreshadows a future interest in thinking of buildings as landscapes

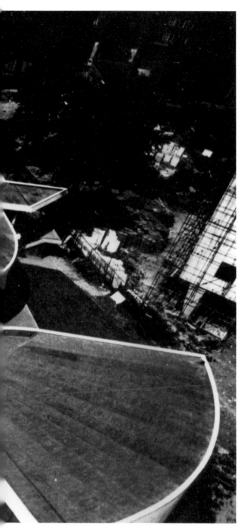

Hallfield School, Paddington, London

In 1954 he designed Keeling House in Bethnal Green, which would become the first local authority tower block to be listed as a building of architectural interest. His idiosyncratic Fitzwilliam College, Cambridge, was completed in 1963. His later works include the imposing University of East Anglia, buildings for the University of London and the European Investment Bank in Luxembourg, and his best-known project, the National Theatre, completed in 1976.

The Royal College of Physicians is on the cusp of this career. Lasdun was a talent not fully proven at the time of his appointment, but with the completion of the building he was established, with a high-profile building to his name. The College is one of his most accomplished works, fusing what until then could be a disparate set of stylistic directions. It is also his most successful – while the National Theatre has provoked hostility as well as praise, on both aesthetic and functional grounds, the College has been largely admired for its entire life and among other things is now listed Grade I.

The College, guided by the architectural historian John Summerson, was taking a gamble, which Lasdun later described as 'a monumental act of faith', when they appointed him and it paid off. As Curtis puts it, it is the work in Lasdun's artistic development 'in which all becomes clear'. With it he 'came to maturity … combining the intellectual and emotional sides of his nature, the organic and classicizing tendencies of his work.'

Like Le Corbusier, Lasdun believed that buildings should take the forms of their own time and exploit twentieth-century construction techniques such as reinforced concrete. Like Le Corbusier he was impressed and inspired by historic and ancient buildings, including Brunelleschi's Pazzi Chapel and the Greek theatre at Epidaurus. He saw the modern movement as a reinvention of architecture, comparable to that which took place in the Renaissance, but not as a rejection of everything that had gone before.

He was not a dogmatist nor an ideologue, neither utopian nor futurist, but believed in designing buildings specific to their situations. 'As a practising architect,' he said, 'I have one foot, perhaps, in the future, but basically I am concerned with the present.' A major influence was *The Architecture of Humanism* of 1914, by the English art historian and poet Geoffrey Scott. As Curtis records, Lasdun often cited a particular passage, which challenges the functionalist idea that structure should govern architectural form:

The art of architecture studies not structure in itself, but the effect of structure on the human spirit. Empirically, by intuition and example, it learns where to discard, where to conceal, where to emphasize, and where to imitate, the facts of construction. It creates, by degrees, a humanized dynamics. For that task, constructive science is a useful slave, and perhaps a useful ally, but certainly a blind master.

He had a particular hero from history in the English baroque architect Nicholas Hawksmoor. Hawksmoor's East London churches, with their massive towers in sepulchral Portland stone, show a freedom of expression and an independence from conventional rules, indeed a positive delight in overturning them. They show how, through a combination of weight and detail, architecture can make dumb minerals communicate emotional force.

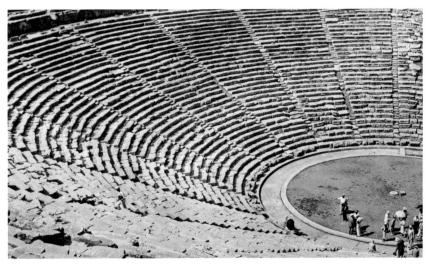

The Greek theatre at Epidavros or Epidaurus

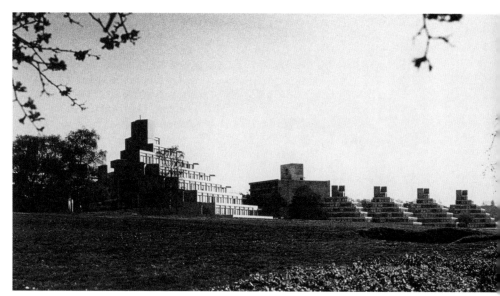

University of East Anglia

Lasdun's transformation of Corbusian modernism included his idea that buildings could resemble landscapes and interact with them. The ziggurats of the University of East Anglia, set in open parkland outside Norwich, embody this idea, and in his later career he developed the concept of 'strata' whereby buildings would be composed of pronounced horizontal layers, of geological inspiration, which would be platforms for human activity.

Alongside his interest in the idea of landscape went one in the realities of cities. Modernist architects of the 1920s sometimes saw existing cities as places to be ignored, or wiped clean, to make way for new creations. Cities, for them, were terminally dysfunctional and unhygienic, but Lasdun was of a generation that began to re-evaluate the inherited fabric within which they worked. 'I cannot,' he said,

> *separate my ideas about architecture from the nature of cities which are there in time, have to change and have to grow, and I really see architecture as a microcosm of the city. Any one building seems to me to be reflecting almost the same sort of activities, the same aspirations, as any piece of the city.*

Thus Keeling House was an attempt to interpret the patterns of East End street life in a vertical structure, while the St James's Place flats aimed to complement the neoclassical architecture of its neighbour Spencer House, without either hostility or mimicry. The Royal College of Physicians would be the most complex and sophisticated of these interrelations of old and new.

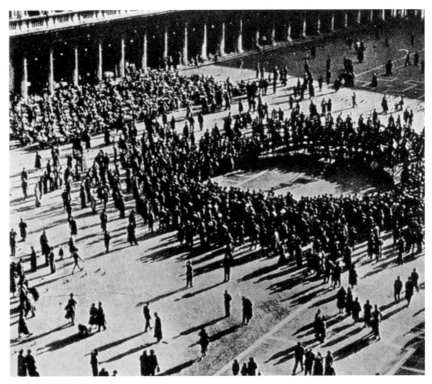

Piazza San Marco, Venice

Perhaps most important to Lasdun was an idea represented by a blown-up photograph which he kept in his office. It showed the Piazza San Marco in Venice as seen from the air, with sections of its famous façades, its paving and a crowd gathering in a circle around some unknown event. The point of the image was that the piazza was not made by buildings alone, but by the interaction of buildings and people. With the National Theatre, for example, Lasdun wanted to create what he called the 'fourth theatre' – in addition to the building's three auditoria he aimed to make a performance space out of its generous foyers and terraces, in which the audience were the players. The purpose of its pronounced strata was to create 'public places, public domains … an extension of the city'.

Lasdun used to tell a story about his wartime experiences in France in which he came across a solitary horse roaming the grounds of a chateau, abandoned by the retreating enemy. Breaking the relevant rules of the British army, he acquired the horse for himself, and it accompanied him on the advance towards Germany. The architect would gallop the animal along the airstrips that he had helped build. This image, of freedom and animation expressed across a horizontal plane, can with hindsight be seen as a premonition of his later work.

PEOPLE AND SPACE

In the Royal College of Physicians, Lasdun could work out his ideas on the interrelation of human activity and built form in complex and specific ways. This was an institution, and therefore a brief and a building, with multiple aspects and patterns of behaviour. Its functions are both symbolic and practical and include research, administration, exhibition, governance, examination, public lectures and ceremonies. Its inhabitants and users include members of the medical professions at every stage of their careers, the staff essential to the working of the institution and the building, and members of the general public attending lectures and events or just wandering through.

The basics of the brief included a library, a lecture theatre, administrative offices, meeting rooms, a dining hall, space for exhibiting the College's paintings and other artefacts, space for receptions and the necessary support, such as kitchens, cloakrooms, circulation space and mechanical plant, to make them work. 'The prime mover' of the interior, said Lasdun, was 'the connexion between the main elements of the plan.' Here his Beaux-Arts training at the AA had its benefits, concerned as it was with the ordering of spaces, especially for ceremonial purposes.

Beyond these uses, the building had to serve an institution which had been in existence since 1518 and occupied four former buildings. It had built up traditions, memories, protocols, habits, rituals, collections, while at the same time changing and renewing. In the earlier locations, for example, anatomical lectures and research took place on site, but from the early nineteenth century such work was carried out elsewhere.

Professional institutions, especially those centuries old, have an inherent conservatism. It is part of their job to maintain the stability and status quo that allows their members to do their work. At the same time, especially in a field where scientific discovery plays an important part, they must move forward and enable progress. Parallel to this tension between past and future is one between seclusion and openness, or priesthood and laity. Professional institutions establish, through examinations and qualifications, necessary barriers which only some people can pass. They protect their knowledge and customs, for good and bad reasons. But they should also serve the public and welcome public involvement.

These tensions are built into the College, and into its building. At the time that Lasdun was appointed, as Barnabas Calder describes, the College was changing its culture, under the presidency of Robert Platt. Platt 'felt that such a learned body had a duty to tell people if they were making themselves ill' and should therefore engage more actively with the public and with public policy. In 1962, for example, he held the first ever press conference at the Royal College of Physicians, to launch the College's hugely influential report on smoking and health.

The College had, since 1825, occupied a handsome Greek revival building in Pall Mall East, on the edge of what would become Trafalgar Square, designed by the British Museum's architect Robert Smirke. It would be fair to call the building, which is now Canada House, clubby: it was on the edge of Clubland and originally housed the Union Club as well as the College. Smirke, who designed the Oxford and Cambridge and Carlton Clubs, gave the building an imposing Ionic portico leading to a grand staircase. It announced its importance and its gentlemanly exclusivity.

The College had been considering leaving Pall Mall East since 1920, for reasons of space, but by the late fifties the move would also be cultural. The new building had somehow to be more open, reflecting Platt's new spirit, while maintaining the dignity of the institution. The appointment of a modernist architect, who by the standards of his slow-maturing profession was on the young side, was a sign of intent.

Successful architects tend to be decisive and confident, or if you like arrogant, in determining what is good for their clients. It is hard for them be otherwise as construction is such a complex process, with so many opinions, interests and hazards, that doubt can be fatal. Serious architects also believe themselves to serve more than the people who are paying their fees. They are designing for the building's users and visitors, for passers-by, and for a future when all involved in a project's making will be dead but the structure will still be there. The invocation of the public and of posterity can be a useful pretext for imposing the architect's artistic will, but these factors are unquestionably significant.

Lasdun was no exception – he had a forceful design personality and his critics called him arrogant. But he also had a genuine interest in the life his buildings would contain. Speaking of his experience with the College, he came up with a formulation which elegantly described an architect's duties and responsibilities to his clients, while also giving himself power to decide what was good for them:

> *our job is to give the client, on time and on cost, not what he wants but what he never dreamed he wanted and, when he gets it, he recognises it as something he wanted all the time.*

As it happened, the College's building was not precisely on time nor on budget, but Lasdun's clients did get the undreamed-of thing they had always wanted. One sign of this success is that the architect remained close to the institution for the rest of his life, becoming an Honorary Fellow in 1975 and being asked to design the extension containing the Council Chamber and Seligman Theatre which, completed in 1998, would be one of his last buildings. Following his death in 2001, his memorial service was held in the College.

This success did not happen by accident. As Calder puts it, 'Lasdun approached the briefing process not as a tedious but necessary enquiry into the number and type of rooms required but as a formative inspiration for his design work.' As the

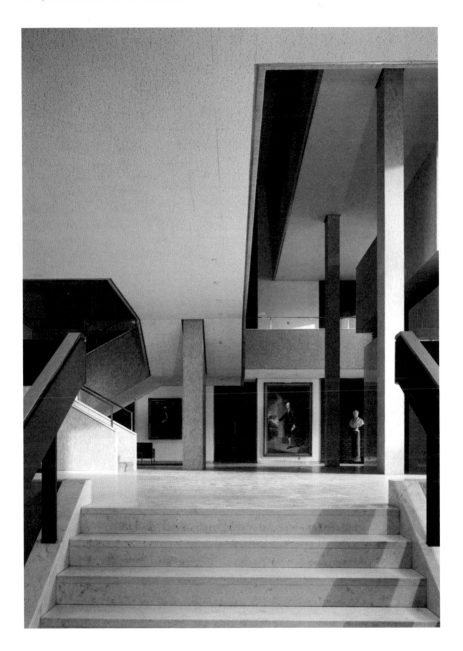

Our job is to give the client . . . not what he wants but what he never dreamed he wanted

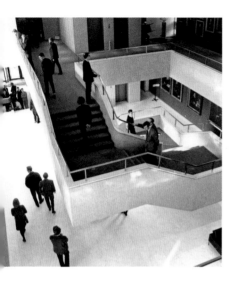

president reported in 1959, the architect was 'taking the greatest care to study the functions, traditions and ceremonies of this old society.' As Lasdun himself described it, he was more interested in what people do than what they say they want. The building which now stands is the product of long and detailed conversations with representatives of the College and of its many activities. It is also a piece of form-making and its architecture exists in the interaction between construction and life.

Much of Lasdun's building is about the play of open and closed. In some ways it is like Smirke's in that it presents a portico to the outside world that, with its almost-windowless planes, forbids as much as it welcomes. As in Smirke's building the portico leads to a grand central stair. Beneath the formal white superstructure, which might be seen as an elevated temple of knowledge, there is, however, a looser, more transparent world. Once you are under the portico, you are embraced by it and you are offered the choice to move forward towards the light, up gradual steps, or turn right to the still-enclosing spaces that lead to the lecture theatre.

In this ninety-degree choice of routes, straight on or right, you are experiencing Platt's concept of the College as interpreted by Lasdun's plan. Platt's belief in engagement meant that the lecture theatre would be placed at the front of the site for ease of public access, with a route which, while sharing the entrance with the whole institution, did not require the laity to travel deep inside.

If you do walk straight ahead you follow a line of spatial contrast (from dark and low to bright and high) into the Marble Hall and then onwards up the central stair to the galleries, libraries and the Osler Room, the venue for official dinners. It is a journey through layers, towards spaces of deeper or higher knowledge and professional definition, that reflects the lifetime ascent of a physician's career.

Much of Lasdun's building is about the play of open and closed. In some ways it is like Smirke's in that it presents a portico to the outside world that, with its almost-windowless planes, forbids as much as it welcomes.

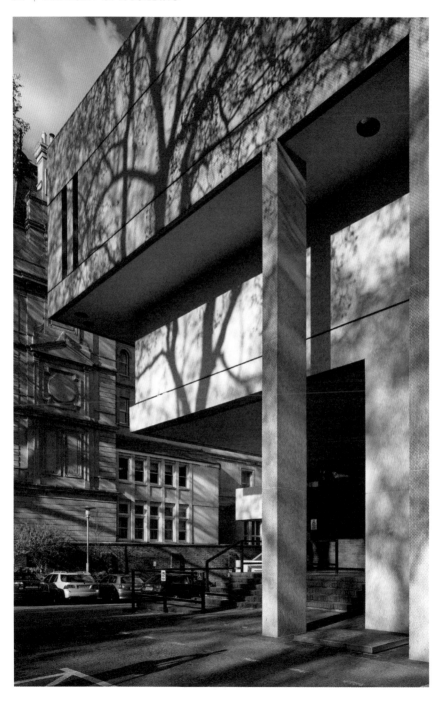

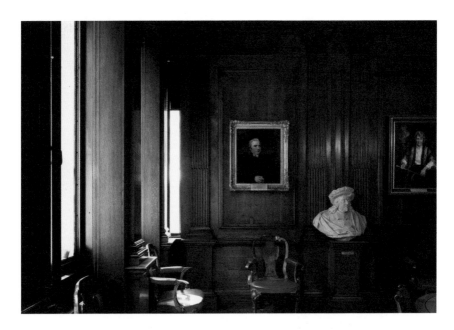

On the right you pass the box containing the Censors' Room, whose interior is lined with the Spanish oak panelling which has followed the College to its different premises since it was first installed in its 1675 building in Warwick Lane. The Censors' Room was the venue of the terrifying interviews which decided if you would become a member of the College – you only got one shot and the outcome would decide the success or failure of the rest of your career. In Lasdun's design the room stands like a guardhouse next to the promise of the staircase. In Calder's view, the arrangement 'dramatises' the moment of acceptance or rejection with the 'life-changing ascension' represented by the stair.

The Censors' Room was the venue of the terrifying interviews which decided if you would become a member of the College – you only got one shot

The Cubist/Paul Klee composition of Hall and garden offers a visual flow in which, although your eye travels easily from inside to out, you cannot move directly from one to the other. The spaces of entry and circulation create a separate physical flow, by turns complementary and contradictory to the visual connections. At times you see a place and can get straight to it, at others you can and you cannot. These combinations of offer and denial are part of an idea of openness that is also complex – some things and places are not as available, or as instantly so, as others.

It is possible to see Lasdun's building as hierarchical. There are the layers of acceptance and enlightenment that you have to penetrate. The building's two main

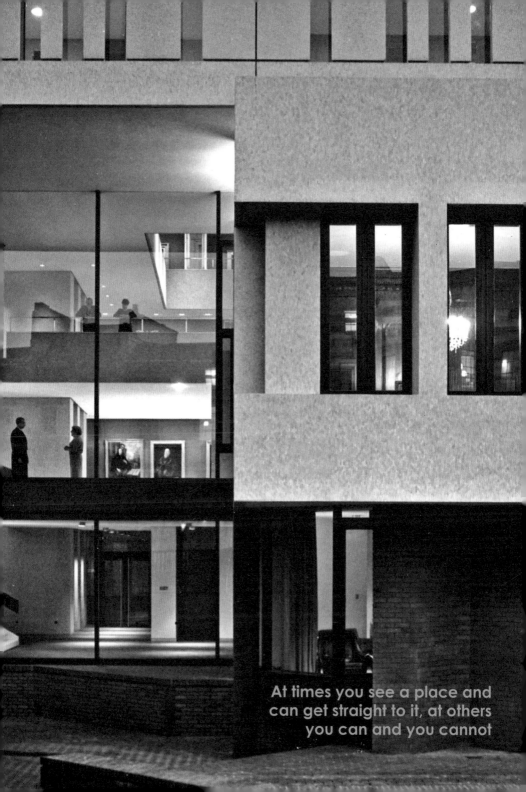

At times you see a place and
can get straight to it, at others
you can and you cannot

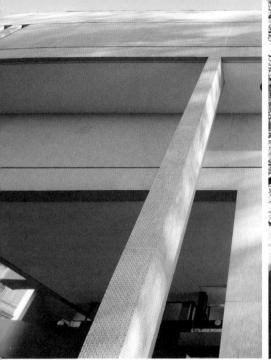
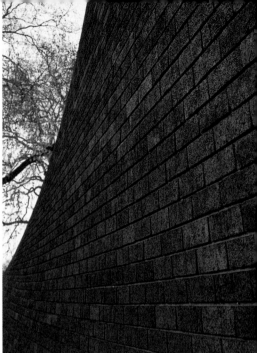

external finishes, Torinese porcelain mosaic in a specially commissioned off-white and blue-black engineering brick from Staffordshire, also seem to code its activities with maximum emphasis. The mosaic, celestial and light, defines the highest, most valued, more exclusive, activities of the College. The dark brick, the stuff of the earth, is used on the publicly accessible lecture theatre and on humbler elements. It reappears on the rear elevation, in impressive but brusque horizontal bands amid the light-stucco nineteenth-century façades of Albany Street, to denote the administrative offices. The same material is used for paving, reinforcing the impression that the brick structures have grown out of the ground.

Mosaic is a material of Byzantine churches, engineering brick that of Midlands factories and one might read this difference as a white/black,Upstairs/Downstairs, Eloi-versus-Morlocks division between the elite and the rest. This reading is most likely when on the Albany Street side, which was always the least loved part of the College's building – for one contemporary critic it was 'a sausage factory'. Basil Spence, the architect of Coventry Cathedral said he was 'unhappy' with it, to which Lasdun said 'I could do nothing about his "unhappiness" and left it at that. I did not wish to change the elevation.'

You can still see why the critics were troubled, but it is also hard to see how a more genteel or domestic façade would have made sense on what is essentially the base of this major institution. To see the building as elitist and exclusive would, more generally, be a perverse description of what you experience when you visit it. What it rather does is to present its contents as exceptional and as deserving respect, but to which the non-specialist visitor can gain access. The severity of the first approach, whether towards the portico or the back, turns out to be the toughest part. After that you feel at no point discouraged or turned away until you get to places that are necessarily private. Once through the glass entrance doors you can go remarkably far before you find another barrier.

The defensive aspects of the exterior make of the inner spaces, in particular the linked pair of the garden and the Marble Hall, a protected, collegiate place. The garden, a living museum of medicinal plants that now contains over 1,300 types and is enclosed by a combination of Lasdun and Nash, has the quality of a cloister or a College court. Lasdun modestly called it 'a small-scale backwater' which nonetheless 'defines in physical terms a scholastic body, inward looking and protected from traffic noise'. As for the Marble Hall, there is after a tough approach something unexpectedly fragile and vulnerable about the way that it opens up to the exterior and about the thin sheets of glass that enclose it.

The uses of the building run from solitary study through everyday office work to grand dinners, and its social encounters from the casual to the formal. Lasdun's design responds to this range of moods, for example by making the Dorchester Library a calm, inward-looking room, with limited views out, and a plain rectangular form that resists the spatial complexities he employed elsewhere. He seems to have derived most pleasure from the opposite, most social end of the scale: by putting the staircase at the centre of the composition, in the abundant space of a triple-height volume, he creates theatre out of the movement of crowds of people. Lasdun liked to say that he was originally asked to produce 'the usual staircase'; his response was to create an unusual one.

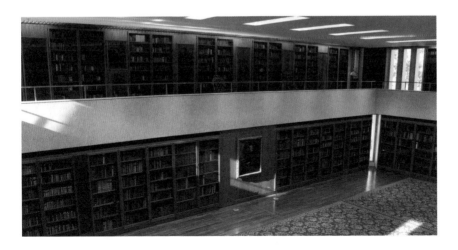

Following the loss of the RCP's library collections during the Great Fire of London, 1666, Henry Pierrepont, Marquess of Dorchester (1607–80) presented his magnificent library to the RCP. He instructed that the collection should never be broken up or sold, the books should remain in the same order, and that the RCP would build a suitable library to house them

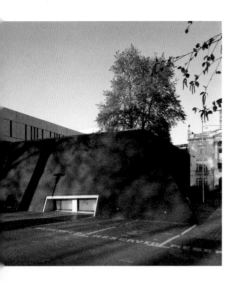

Also vital to the social and ceremonial roles of the College are the Osler Room and Long Rooms, the first a high-ceilinged hall with galleries on two sides, where members and guests can dine in the presence of ancestral portraits. The second, which has good views out, was originally a space for pre-dinner drinks, and both now house, among other things, display events, careers fairs, lunch for delegates, staff meetings, and the staff Christmas party. The Osler and Long Rooms are separated by a wall, which with hydraulic power can rise out of the way, allowing the two to be used as one.

Somewhere between ceremonial and study, and having aspects of both, is the lecture theatre. It is placed near the entrance as something to which the general public would frequently be invited, whereas the Osler Room is buried quite deep in the building. The theatre announces itself, if enigmatically, as the brick mound which you first encounter when approaching the building. Nowadays architects like to symbolise public accessibility with expanses of glass, but Lasdun chose only to hint at the theatre's purpose: its shape is an external expression of its internal nature as an auditorium, in a quietened-down version of a device that Russian Constructivist architects liked to use.

It is unusual for a building to be as varied in its uses as the Royal College and this variety was an inspiration to Lasdun. He responded with an equal range of spaces – open, intimate, grand, light, dark, introvert, public, low, high – which might be typified by the building's staircases. As well as the grand affair at the centre of the Marble Hall, there is the spiral, enclosing, castle-like and a little mysterious, which descends from the foyer of the Wolfson Theatre to the cloakroom and toilets at lower ground floor level. There is also the stair that serves the office accommodation, functional but still dignified. Each of these three stairs has a distinct character and mood, reflecting its respective role, but each feels like an integral part of the whole.

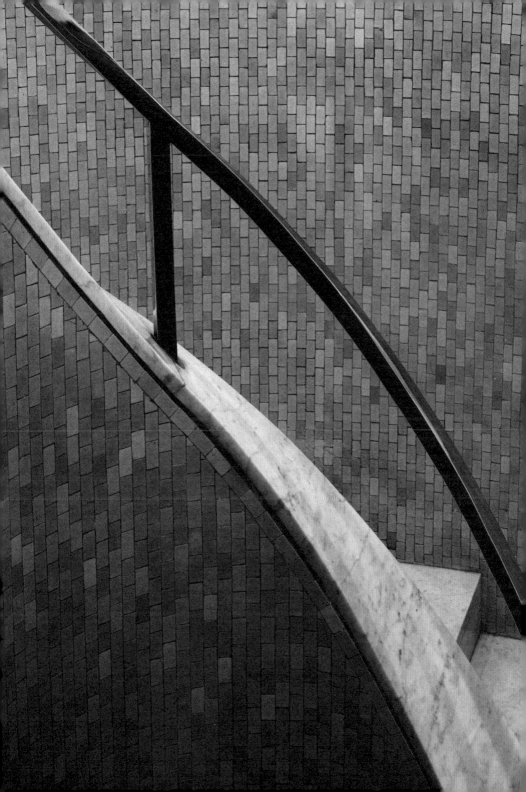

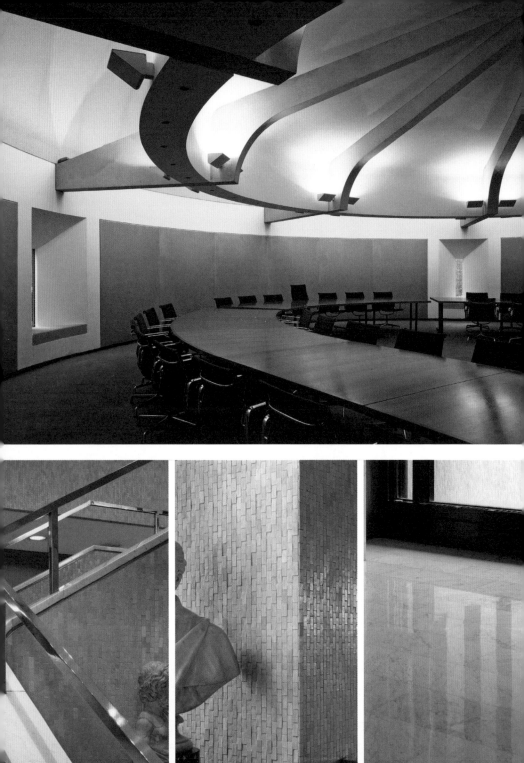

The 1990s addition adds further to the College's range of moods. In this two-storey structure Lasdun reprises his theme of placing light above dark, with the luminous Council Chamber resting on the cavernous Seligman Theatre, but the addition's circular geometry brought something new to the complex. With its ribbed ceiling and suggestions of a monastic chapter house, the Council Chamber also brings Gothic references to what was previously mostly classical.

In all this multiplicity the building as a whole retains its coherence, such that many of its effects come through the play of diversity and order. Detail and finish play a crucial role, with the exterior duality of light and dark taken inside and then adjusted. The external mosaic and brick continue and marble is added, enhancing the sense that the entrance and the Marble Hall are at least partly outdoor in spirit. At the same time the palette is enriched and (slightly) softened with bronze, brass, wall fabrics, oak, an east African hardwood called muninga and carpet in a colour sometimes called 'golden' but which Lasdun always referred to as 'ginger'. Finally, in the offices, more humdrum plaster and suspended ceilings take over.

Sensuality is added to this rigorous building by subtle touches, neither easy nor cheap to achieve, like marble on the inner balustrade of the main stair that curves and twists as it rises. Both material and detail are tuned to suit different spaces (with timber being used extensively, for example, on the walls and floors of the Dorchester Library) but also to sustain the overall intent of the design. 'Detailing,' said Lasdun, 'is not a question of whether a thing is rough, smooth, shiny or matt. It is concerned with the intellectual texture of the whole design and its consistency.'

It is, as Calder points out, a highly crafted building, with elements such as the sloping, irregularly curving brick wall of the Wolfson Theatre requiring a high degree of skill. The absence of frame where large glass sheets hit walls or ceiling is crucial to the flow of inside and out, and the positioning of ventilation grilles and recessed lights could, wrongly handled, have been fatal. As Le Corbusier told Maxwell Fry, as reported by Lasdun, the difference between good and bad architecture 'is a matter of centimetres'.

> The difference between good and bad architecture 'is a matter of centimetres'

The diversity of materials and details in the Royal College of Physicians is exceptional in Lasdun's own work, in modernist architecture and in the more assertive versions of modernism of the late 1950s and early 1960s. By the standards of the latter, they would have seemed luxurious, going on decadent. The building is singular, a one-off, designed at a time when architects were striving to find universal, repeatable solutions, on which point Lasdun could be a little defensive. But its multiplicity and richness reflects that of the lives it was to contain and also the dignity which the Royal College of Physicians would have felt proper to itself. At the same time it is not pompous nor pretentious. In almost all its decisions, the design remains alert and purposeful.

The reciprocity of people and space is a large part of Lasdun's intent (as he said, 'this kind of space needs people') and an essential factor in the building's success. Since it was completed, it has become much more intensively used, with external bodies holding talks and receptions, to which added demands it has responded with grace.

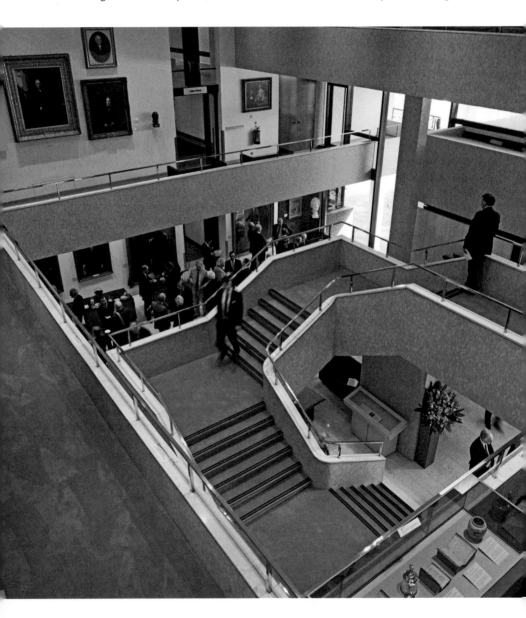

TIME

Herbert Baker (1862–1946) was a prolific and successful architect but one on whom history, when it remembers him at all, does not look kindly. He ravaged John Soane's masterpiece, the Bank of England, and tampered with Edwin Lutyens' grand vision for New Delhi. 'I met my Bakerloo' was the latter's comment on the experience. Baker practised a version of classicism that was respectable but often tepid and backward looking.

He designed South Africa House, on the opposite side of Trafalgar Square from the Royal College of Physicians' previous home in what is now Canada House. When Lasdun was being assessed as a prospective architect of the College's new building, one of his interviewers pointed out of the window at Baker's work and asked if Lasdun would design something like that. The answer was 'no' which, as the College had already decided they wanted a modern architect, was the right one.

Most architecture engages with and reacts to its past, but in the twentieth century this relationship became fraught. Modern movement architects believed that science and industry had made a world unlike anything before and therefore required a new kind of architecture, while remaining in thrall to the classical tradition.

Critics of modernism accused it of indifference to the past when in fact the preoccupation was almost too great. What is true is that modern movement architects avoided, as if it were an infectious disease, the explicit use of ornamental detail derived from historic buildings. They preferred to learn more abstractly from precedents, in areas such as composition, proportion and form.

Thus, while you won't find a dentil or a cornice on the College's building, still less a scroll or an acanthus leaf, there is latent in its white superstructure the form of a classical temple. It is symmetrical, rectangular and aspires to be freestanding as it emerges from the looser gaggle of subsidiary structures at ground level. It has columns which support an upper level which might be thought an entablature, which even has traces of the triglyphs of the Doric order, suggested by the pattern of vertical slits on the top floor. There is also, in the combination of brick and mosaic, a reinterpretation of the combinations of base and superstructure, or of rustication and refinement, with which classical architecture defines the below and the above.

This, however, is an idea of temple which has undergone transformations. It has firstly been filtered through Le Corbusier's Villa Savoye in Poissy of 1928–31, which translated classical columns into *pilotis* – 'pilings' or 'piers' – slender cylinders of reinforced concrete rather than marble. At the Villa Savoye, whose aesthetic is shaped by the clean lines of cars and ships, the horizontal is stressed to a degree you don't find in conventionally classical buildings.

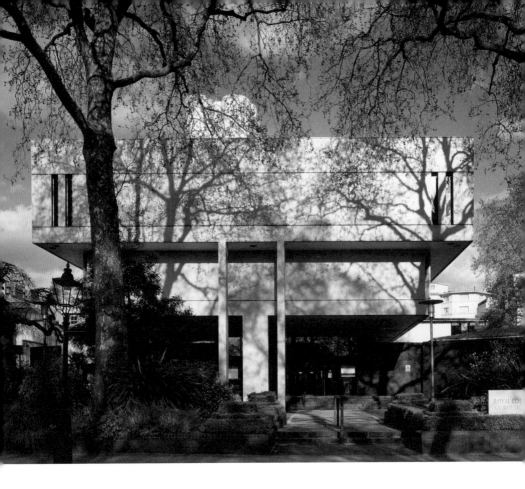

It is also possible to see the influences of Hawksmoor and Brunelleschi. The portico presents a blank, frontal aspect, which echoes both the former's Christ Church Spitalfields and the latter's Pazzi Chapel, and creates a series of layers through which the entering visitor has to pass

The College also has something ship-like about it, and its edges sometimes the sharp precision of the machine, but Lasdun takes Le Corbusier's adaptations further. At the front, the skinniness of the uprights is taken to the point where it seems impossible that they can hold anything much up, and they are removed from the corners, which is where classical architecture likes to add emphasis and strength. The quasi-entablature has gone in the opposite direction, towards heft and breadth, to create a strikingly and deliberately top-heavy composition. These mannerisms caused the great critic and historian Sir Nikolaus Pevsner to call the College 'post-modern'. It was one of the very first applications of the term to architecture and it wasn't meant as a compliment.

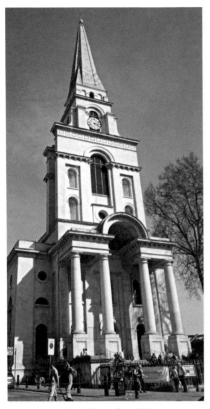

Hawksmoor's Christ Church Spitalfields

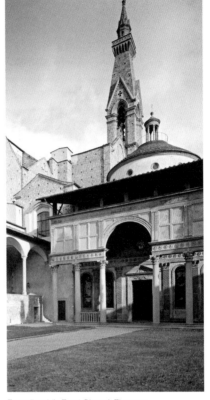

Brunelleschi's Pazzi Chapel, Florence

It is also possible to see the influences, again abstracted, of Lasdun's heroes Hawksmoor and Brunelleschi. The portico presents a blank, frontal aspect, which echoes both the former's Christ Church Spitalfields and the latter's Pazzi Chapel, and creates a series of layers through which the entering visitor has to pass. As in both these works mass is combined with lines thinly incised in the surfaces, making the building look weighty and papery at once.

The building's most immediate engagement with architectural history is with the terraces designed by John Nash, or by others in modified versions of his style, that make up its near surroundings. Built as speculative developments, as part of Nash's creation of Regent's Park from 1811 onwards, these are brick buildings with elevations of painted stucco. As in developers' architecture before and since, there are elements of pretension and deception in these buildings: the stucco was a cheap way to look like stone and terraces were embellished with grandiose columns and pilasters. They were composed in such a way, with porticoes and corner pavilions, that several homes would collectively resemble the façade of a single country house.

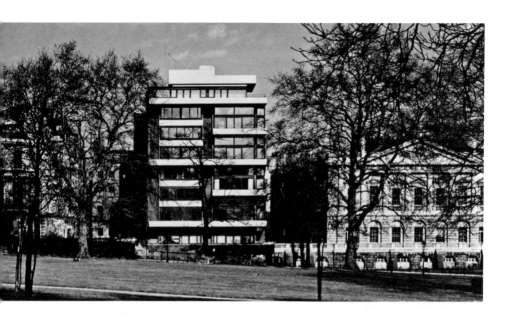

The building for the Royal College echoes Nash in its whitish tone, its similar parapet height and its latent classicism, then contrasts through its modernity and its inversions

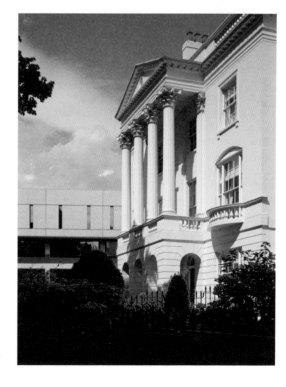

ABOVE: 26 St James's Place, London
RIGHT: 9–10 St Andrews Place, now William Harvey House, the Royal College of Physicians' member and fellow accommodation

These façades are partly stage sets that create a theatre of palatial grandeur not entirely supported by the reality of the buildings behind them.

Even so, and despite the fact that poor construction has often necessitated comprehensive rebuilding, Nash's work around Regent's Park has come to be counted among the greatest of Britain's urban set pieces and among the outstanding examples of the country's domestic architecture. It demands a serious response from any architect not completely insensitive. Lasdun's was to engage respectfully but vigorously with his predecessor.

Here he was building on his work on the block of flats at 26 St James's Place, designed but not built at the time that he won the Royal College commission. This also faces a royal park and has distinguished architecture for a neighbour, John Vardy's Spencer House of 1756–66, which is now described as 'one of the most ambitious aristocratic town houses ever built in London' and 'the city's only great eighteenth-century private palace to survive intact'. Here Lasdun designed something which is everything the older building is not – a vertical outline with strong horizontal accents, whereas Spencer House is the opposite, with a staggered rhythm of cantilevered concrete balconies rather than the stone Doric half columns of the Palladian neighbour. Yet, somehow, there is a rapport between the two, coming from echoes in their scale and proportion and a robust confidence common to both.

The building for the Royal College echoes Nash in its whitish tone, its similar parapet height and its latent classicism, then contrasts through its modernity and its inversions. It differs through its solidity and structural integrity: where Nash offered stucco illusions, Lasdun created a well-made building whose structure is visible. Then, having established both similarity and difference, he got his new building to work with the old ones to enclose the garden. Finally, through the use of glass, he created a play of new and old that could be experienced from the interior, in which the elevation of St Andrews Place becomes a deferred fourth wall for the Marble Hall.

If architectural history is one way in which the building engages with time, there is also the span of the institution itself, now approaching half a millennium. The Lasdun building is its fifth home, meaning that the College moves on average about once a century, from the time that it occupied the house of its founder, Thomas Linacre, close to St Paul's Cathedral. The College took two rooms of the Stone House, as it was called, with a theatre for anatomical lectures added later.

In 1614 the growth of the College led to its move to another house, also near St Paul's, at Amen Corner, a double-fronted but still quite homely looking structure which would be destroyed in the Great Fire of 1666. The successor, designed by the scientist and architect Robert Hooke and completed in 1675, was a leap in scale and architectural ambition: it was no longer domestic but collegiate or institutional, with a formal court, a pedimented elevation and an educated classical style. It included an oak-panelled public gallery called the

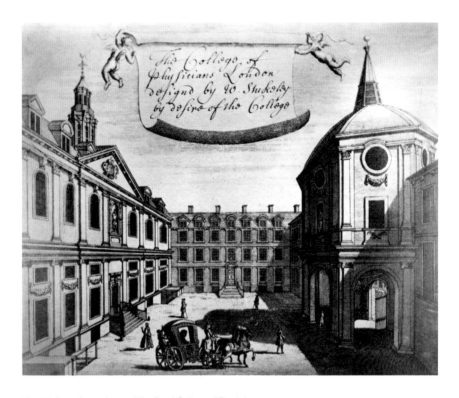

Warwick Lane, former home of the Royal College of Physicians

Great Room and a domed polygonal structure containing the anatomy theatre which, perched on arches above the entrance to the court, must have been one of the most intriguing structures of its time. A library, by another scientist-architect Christopher Wren, was added later.

Like its predecessors the third building was close to St Paul's, in Warwick Lane, and it attracted generous donations from city merchants and other sources. For the first time it presented the College both as a dignified, important and self-aware institution, and as a place that addressed and sometimes welcomed the public in. In use for 150 years, it was the longest-lived, so far, of the College's homes and it set the pattern for its successors by Smirke and Lasdun.

The move to Pall Mall East in 1825 reflected a desire to leave an area that John Evelyn had described as 'so obscure a hole' and to follow the shift of public life and society away from the City of London. The location of the new building was part of an area then being comprehensively remodelled, including the creation of what would become Trafalgar Square on the site of former royal stables. The National Gallery, by William Wilkins, would be built next door to the new College, shortly after its completion.

With this move, practical medicine was no longer carried out on the College's premises: there was now no anatomy theatre or laboratory on site. Rather, as noted above, Smirke's building had some of the qualities of a club. It later became Canada House, the home of that country's High Commission, and its grand-but-not-excessive architecture is well suited to representing a nation.

With its move from building to building, on an ascending scale of size and prestige, the College gathered both rituals (as described above) and belongings. William Harvey, for example, donated his personal collections in 1654, only for many of them to be destroyed in 1666. In 1680 the Marquis of Dorchester donated the collection of books that is now housed in the Library that bears his name. Busts and portraits – including one of Harvey saved from the fire – have accumulated over time and are now on show in the Marble Hall and others of the more public spaces.

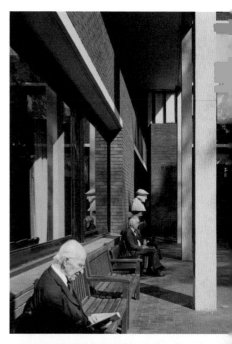

Lasdun's building, consciously or not, has echoes of the grander of its predecessors (though there is not much similarity to the two domestic buildings that the College first occupied). As well as the reconstructed Censors' Room and the radical reinterpretations of Smirke's portico and grand stair, there is a distant affinity in the current building's half-enclosed garden with the court of Hooke's building.

Lasdun also took seriously the display of the inherited artefacts (even if he disrespectfully called them 'the clobber of ancestral memories') not only making space available for them, but considering their placement. By the door at the rear of the Marble Hall, a portrait of Edward Archer, the eighteenth-century pioneer of the treatment of smallpox, makes a welcoming gesture, as if encouraging you on. (Early photos show him in this position, and he is still there.) The heights of the balconies on the Marble Hall are critical – if they were a few inches lower, the larger paintings would not fit.

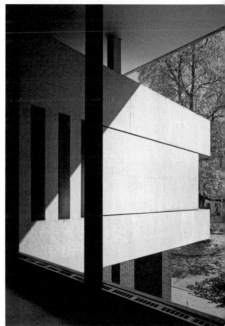

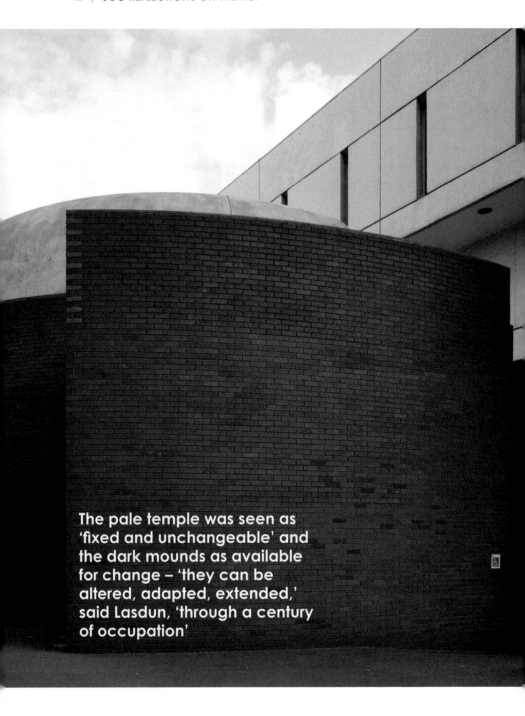

The pale temple was seen as 'fixed and unchangeable' and the dark mounds as available for change – 'they can be altered, adapted, extended,' said Lasdun, 'through a century of occupation'

As with his approach to architectural history, Lasdun makes both connections and discontinuities between the modern and the past. The Censors' Room sits well in a structure that its seventeenth-century makers could not have dreamt of, but at the room's corners Lasdun interrupts the panelling with narrow windows, which is his way of reminding you that the twentieth century is also there. Inside the Censors' Room the gold-framed oil paintings sit comfortably against their oak backgrounds; in some other parts of the College they are put into a more contrasting relationship with the Corbusian forms.

Then, alongside timescales measured in centuries, there are those of decades, years, months and days, for example the adaptation and growth of the building in response to the development of the institution it houses. Lasdun represented such change through his contrast between mosaic and brick – the pale temple being seen as 'fixed and unchangeable' and the dark mounds as available for change – 'they can be altered, adapted, extended,' said Lasdun, 'through a century of occupation'. Here he anticipates the high-tech architecture of the next decade, in particular Piano and Rogers' Pompidou Centre, which also wanted to differentiate the fixed and changing parts of a building. As with the latter the intent is partly symbolic, as it would not actually make much sense to rearrange the sculpted, crafted form of the Wolfson Theatre. But the deft insertion, in the 1990s, of the new structure containing the council chamber and the Seligman theatre, vindicates Lasdun's initial concept. A substantial addition, the domed circular form was something else again from the original

building's range of motifs, could be made without disrupting the clarity of its architectural idea.

There is also the ageing of the building, a more subtle affair than on Lasdun's other works. On the National Theatre and other buildings the architect liked to expose raw concrete, often imprinted with the grain of the boards used in its formwork, which would then weather dramatically. It was a feature often criticised, but robustly defended by the architect. He made an analogy with the face of a person: if it gets dirty, you should wash it, but to change with time is honourable and inevitable.

With the Royal College the extensive use of exposed concrete is limited and the mosaic used instead, well maintained, still looks almost as new. Your sense that this is not a brand new building comes from a faint mellowing of the mosaic, its grout, and the brick, and some background awareness that these were materials more of the 1960s than now. Such concrete as there is would also have aged more markedly, until it was painted in the 1990s.

Lasdun's orchestration of relationships to the building's natural surroundings, his selective opening-up and closing-down of views, creates a particular awareness of seasonal rhythms, while the building's multiple light sources allow the changing weather to register inside – as slabs and shards of sunshine, or as a soft, cloudy light on a dull day. Inside and out, the undecorated planes of the modernist style allow shadows to read, both clean-cut shapes cast on itself by the building's own projections and the lighter patterns of leaves or winter branches.

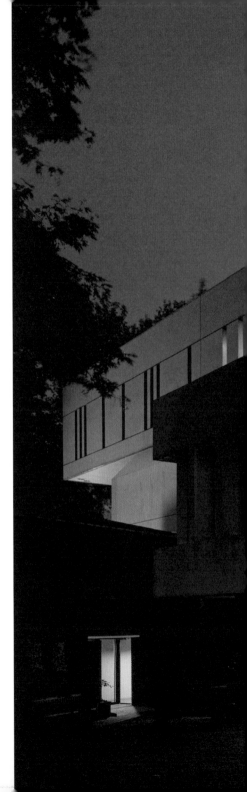

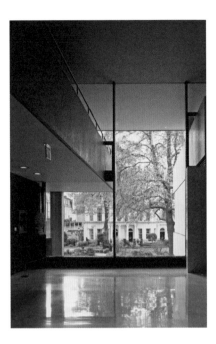

At night, with the heavy superstructure floating on internal illumination, the building becomes something else again. Photographers of the building, throughout its life, have been keen on picking up its effects of fluctuating light.

To these rhythms of history and nature can be added the daily patterns of inhabitation and use, practical, studious, social and ceremonial, individual and collective, purposeful and wandering. Of course, all buildings exist in time and change with weather and use. The point is whether they deny or ignore these properties or welcome them and allow them to enrich the architecture. The College does the latter.

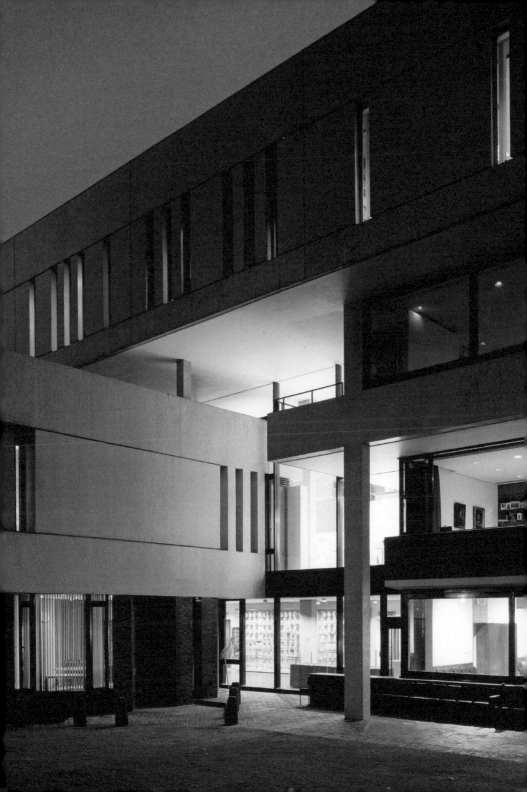

COMPLEXITY AND CONTRADICTION

As well as the imagery of building as body, there is another set of analogies between the make-up of a human being and of architecture. This is the realm of emotion – the extent to which arrangements of spaces and inanimate construction materials might express, reflect, communicate or complement human feelings. Buildings are said to have 'characters' or 'moods', sometimes 'personalities'. They can be called gloomy, arrogant, witty, playful, charming, brooding, pompous, self-effacing.

As in human psychology, buildings can be perverse, paradoxical or contradictory. What they claim to be, and what they are, might be different. Their apparent and actual intentions might diverge, or they might embody multiple desires that cannot be reconciled. They might include such things as fear, pessimism, darkness and conflict, although architecture has more difficulty expressing such things than other art forms. Artists and writers might be celebrated for engaging with dangerous emotions, but it is hard for an architect to persuade a client to spend millions on an essay on alienation or despair. Architects are under pressure to be optimistic.

To discuss emotion in architecture is also to raise the question of whose feelings we are speaking – the architect's, the client's, the inhabitants' or users'? All ultimately make what a building is, and architecture acts as an intermediate term between the desire of those who make it and the experience of those who use it. In other words it communicates, powerfully but clumsily, between people who often don't know each other. This fact gives rise to the well-known gripe about architects, that they impose their dreams and fantasies on others. At the same time, attempts by architects to be neutral or self-effacing also tend to fail, it being hard to escape the fact that, no matter what, almost any building is a significant intervention in people's lives. The best architecture consists of propositions – well-considered, imaginative ideas about what the future might be, carried out with skill and conviction, while also allowing and encouraging the possibility that its users will make it into something that its makers hadn't quite conceived.

Denys Lasdun was an architect who designed from his gut and his heart. He could be insightful and articulate and was more literate and cultured than many in his profession, but he was not a rationalist nor a theoretician. He recognised that there was a point beyond which an architect has to rely on instinct, that it is counter-productive to reduce every decision by explanation and analysis. 'Architecture,' he said, 'oscillates between reason and feeling.' Nor, for him, was the process of design about cool calculation:

You have to come to our office and hear the infighting, the differences of opinion, experience the rhythm of design, see how the discipline of architecture has the miraculous power of reconciling differences between young people, middle people and old people. We are not a happy little band who go around agreeing about every problem we are working on. We argue, discuss and absorb information from many different skills.

He belonged to a period when the earlier versions of the modern movement were being questioned as overly mechanistic in trying to apply supposedly scientific methods and industrial construction techniques to the design of habitation. The shift was personified in the career of Le Corbusier. It would be wrong ever to describe him as purely rational or functionalist, but in his earlier work he would sometimes claim that his proposals for cities of towers were driven by efficiency and logic, and that buildings could resemble machines. In later works, such as his chapel in Ronchamp of 1954, his use of curving and irregular forms, and primitive as well as modern building methods, removed any doubt that something other than reason was a motivating factor.

In Britain the modern movement had arrived late, mostly in the form of 1930s private houses and Lubetkin's zoo buildings. It only really took hold after the war as the style of schools, housing and hospitals demanded by Attlee's welfare state. It was given further impetus by the Festival of Britain of 1951, only to prompt a reaction additional to that against the cold functionalism of early modern architecture: the style exemplified by the Royal Festival Hall was seen as too tepid, too compromised, too nice. In the 1950s architects like Alison and Peter Smithson promoted an approach in which, as Alison Smithson put it, the structure of a building would be 'exposed entirely, without interior finishes wherever practicable'. They favoured more robust forms

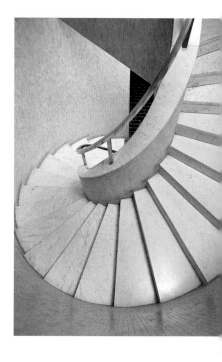

Buildings are said to have 'characters' or 'moods', sometimes 'personalities'. They can be called gloomy, arrogant, witty, playful, charming, brooding, pompous, self-effacing

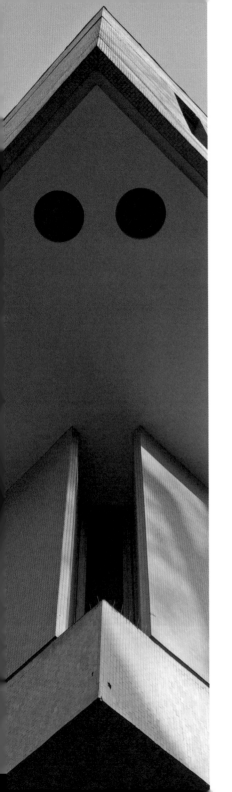

and rougher surfaces and drew on the motifs of Le Corbusier's later works. They liked things to be 'as found' – whether the inherent qualities of building materials or the imperfect conditions of city streets.

In parallel with the contemporary Angry Young Men in theatre, they wanted to provoke, unsettle and challenge complacency. Supported by the critic Reyner Banham they acquired the label 'the New Brutalism', which has a variety of origins: that Peter Smithson's nickname was Brutus was one of them, another that the concrete they liked is called *beton brut* in French. The suggestion of toughness was part of the name's attraction, but it easily became a stick with which to beat the protagonists – they were 'brutalist' and therefore brutal. Recently the writers Jonathan Meades and Owen Hatherley have championed this period, many of whose monuments are disappearing, and used the term 'brutalist' without apology. It is still a hard sell to the general public.

The expressiveness of Brutalism was upsetting to Nikolaus Pevsner, the most influential historian and theorist of his time, who since the 1930s had been campaigning for what he called 'the architecture of reason and functionalism'. Of Ronchamp he wrote, 'woe to him who succumbs to the temptation of reproducing the same effect in another building less isolated … less exceptional in function.' Writing in 1960, at the time Lasdun was working on the College, he wrote that 'we are surrounded once again by freaks and fantasists', by which he referred to the Brutalists but also more generally to the architectural scene of the time.

Lasdun always made it clear that he was not himself a Brutalist and in 1957 he criticised the movement for an attachment to 'formulations' which 'tend to rigidity'. If he followed Geoffrey Scott in believing that structure should be manipulated for its effect 'on the human spirit', this emphasises different values from Alison

Smithson's preference for exposing it at all costs. Nor was the Royal College of Physicians, a building for an ancient institution on the edge of a royal park, the kind of gritty urban project that most appealed to Brutalists.

But he shared some of their preferences – strong forms, rough surfaces, interest in the city as found – which would cause some favourable critics to group Lasdun with the Brutalists, while hostile critics would be happy to use the label against him. In Pevsner's terms, Lasdun would have been more in the category of fantasist than functionalist. Pevsner's biographer Susie Harris writes that the two had 'a bumpy relationship, disrupted by a series of fallings-out, but held together in the end by mutual respect'. She quotes a 1967 letter by Pevsner who, after telling Lasdun that 'you are the most generous of men', asserted that there should be 'no truce' between them. Instead there should be:

> *just agreement that you are*
> *one person and I am another,*
> *both passionately believing in*
> *something worth believing in. I*
> *know, however, that I am stuck,*
> *and you must know that you can*
> *be carried away. If there is one*
> *architect in England today … who*
> *should have his way even where he*
> *overshoots, it's you.*

Pevsner, in other words, did not approve but he felt compelled to admire.

If modernism might, crudely speaking, be split between rationalist and expressive tendencies, there is a comparable split between the orderly and the romantic in English architectural

traditions, exemplified by the difference between the calm Palladianism that took hold in the first quarter of the eighteenth century and its immediate predecessor – inventive, tumultuous, to its critics wayward and excessive – what is now called the English Baroque. Again it is clear on which side Lasdun falls, his hero Hawksmoor being one of the inventive and tumultuous ones. The exterior of the College, with its advances and recessions and the bold and different profiles it presents when approached from different directions, has clear affinities with the drama of Hawksmoor's silhouettes.

Occasionally Lasdun's inventions could be downright peculiar, like the surprised-looking Moorish vaults at Fitzwilliam College, which he teamed with dour brown brick, green copper, slit windows and a portico in the form of a flying triangle of concrete. If his later work looks confident and resolved, these qualities were not achieved without struggle, dead ends and diversions. The College itself has a striking and potentially disparate range of motifs, some of them close to eccentric – slit windows again, the brick mound, the decision to build something resembling a ziggurat on its head.

They hang together more convincingly than at Fitzwilliam, but the resolution is not and does not want to be smooth. There is nervous energy in the vertical slits, in the erosion of corners, and the way the brittle uprights in front of the entrance look inadequate for the load they are carrying. Sometimes, says Calder, 'Lasdun fights his materials', requiring brick and marble to take on shapes that don't come easily to them and require 'remarkable labour' to achieve. The building's plays of offer and denial are there from the first approach: it presents blankness on its front elevation, accentuated by the way that pairs of slit windows are pushed to edges, the welcome of its entrance being something that has to be discovered. And, while the symmetry of its portico suggests a frontal approach, the main routes to it are either oblique or off-centre.

There are other ambiguities and inversions, such as that the building at times looks to be completely freestanding and at others enmeshed with its neighbours – its identity is sometimes graspable and sometimes not. The placing of white mosaic above dark brick makes sense as part of a progression from ground to sky, but it also turns upside-down the pattern of similar tones on the Nash buildings, where the dark slate surmounts the white stucco. Some of these effects were not easily realised: for example the absence of supports at the corners of the portico required demanding and probably expensive cantilevers, with plenty of steel reinforcement. It would have been easier just to prop them with some additional pillars, but less powerful.

If some kind of balance and peace is eventually to be found in the Marble Hall, it is hard achieved, and even here the placing of the stair puts movement at its centre. Throughout the building there is a never-quite-resolved tension between restlessness and repose. The dominant quality is, however, calm, which one arguably appreciates all the more for awareness that it might – but doesn't – dissolve into nervousness. It would be

a mistake to over-analyse the meaning of Lasdun's paradoxes, to ask for example the precise significance of his habit of denying and then yielding. The fact that not everything is as you might expect nonetheless imparts a sense of intellectual and creative energy, that struggle is a part of achievement.

Lasdun's strength of character didn't endear him to everyone and when the reaction set in against the architecture of his period, he bore the brunt of criticism. The National Theatre, for example, would be compared to a nuclear power station. But without that strength of character the College would be a duller place. It imparts a consciousness, a self-awareness as you move through the spaces. As you ascend the few steps between the entrance and the Marble Hall, go from dark to light, or turn to take in a view, these actions are given a different character by a distinctive intelligence built into the fabric and the spaces of the building. Which intelligence, for this writer at least, is neither oppressive nor overly controlling nor intrusive – as Lasdun put it 'the great art of architecture is the art of concealing the art of architecture'.

The relationship of architecture to the actions and emotions for which it is the setting is reciprocal and complementary, not imitative. A building is one thing, humanity another, and you no more need a room to resemble its living contents than you would need to eat chicken off a chicken-shaped plate – difference is an essential part of the relationship. But neither do you want indifference, the feeling that nobody cares about the way one part of the space joins another, how the light falls, or how you are supposed to occupy it.

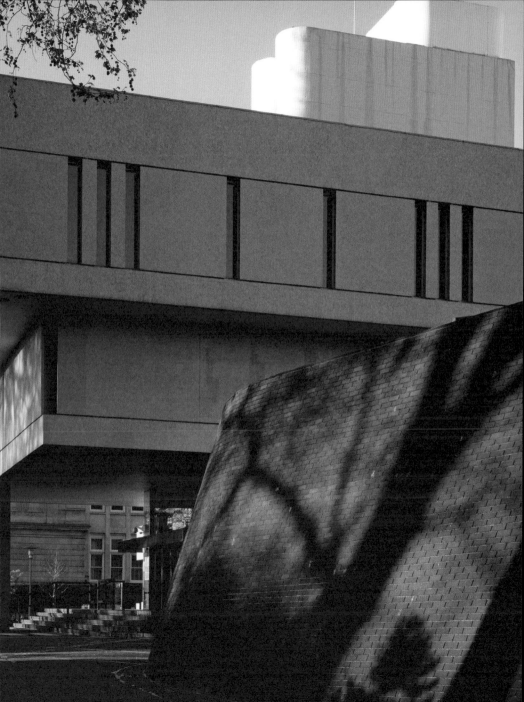

BACK TO THE BODY

I am in a handsome room on the *piano nobile* of the building, just off Harley Street, that was once occupied by the practice of Lasdun Redhouse and Softley. Lasdun, who I know through a family connection, has kindly invited me to lunch so that he can review the scribblings I have produced as a student architect. This being the time when modernism was profoundly out of fashion, I am striving to uncover some alternative.

He looks on with bewilderment, not to say dismay and exasperation. Eventually he feels the need to explain the concept of coherence in architecture and with a thick pencil sketches a human form. It is a version of Vitruvian Man or Le Modulor. This is Rowan Moore, he says, and he circles the head and heart and, delicately pausing before his native frankness takes over, the groin. He goes on to argue that the body has its distinct and vital centres, which at the same time form part of a whole, and that a building should be likewise.

Of his building for the Royal College of Physicians he said, in a talk soon after its completion:

> *This is by no means a perfect building – that would be boring. In fact, it seems to me, looking at it, that it ceases to be a building with a capital 'B'. It is more a piece of organization sensitized to its external context and capable of growth and change. It is, therefore, an organism in which the architect is primarily concerned with routes, focal points and enclosing fabric.*

The use of the word 'organism' is not accidental, but reinforced by other comments in the same lecture. Lasdun speaks of the central hall as the 'belly of the building', and says that, as you ascend the central stair, 'the whole anatomy of the building is made visually clear'. As William Curtis wrote, 'the relevance of his interest in biological analogies did not pass Lasdun by when it came to designing the headquarters of a medical body.' It is also a building to be experienced *with* the body, which reveals itself only by motion through its spaces and up its stairs – it requires an active engagement from its users.

Pushed too far, the image of building-as-body could become banal, especially in the presence of professionals engaged with the intricacy and wonders of the real thing. It is rather one of several layers of intent that collectively make the building what it is. The bodily qualities of the building play an important role in giving form to what, with its multiplicity of shapes, materials, motifs and uses, might otherwise be chaotic. It might have been a bag of bones, but is not.

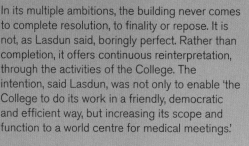

In its multiple ambitions, the building never comes to complete resolution, to finality or repose. It is not, as Lasdun said, boringly perfect. Rather than completion, it offers continuous reinterpretation, through the activities of the College. The intention, said Lasdun, was not only to enable 'the College to do its work in a friendly, democratic and efficient way, but increasing its scope and function to a world centre for medical meetings.'

Shortly after completion he also recalled that 'the decision to commission a modern building was taken over five years ago in a mixed spirit of trepidation and un-enthusiasm. The clients are now said to be won over because the organism ticks – it works.' It still does.

The decision to commission a modern building was taken over five years ago in a mixed spirit of trepidation and un-enthusiasm. The clients are now won over because the organism ticks – it works

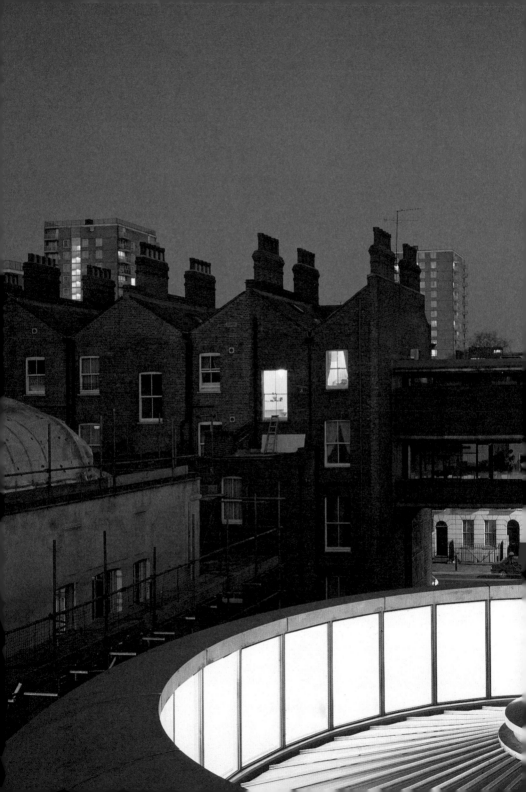

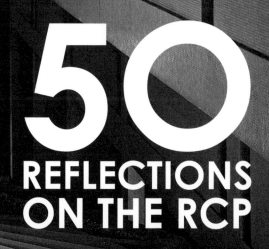

PEOPLE

DENYS LASDUN

Denys Lasdun (1914–2001) was one of the most significant British architects of the second half of the twentieth century. He was a firm believer in the principles of the modern movement and was deeply impressed by Le Corbusier's work, but he transformed these influences into a powerful and individual approach to architecture.

The critic Diana Rowntree, in her obituary of Lasdun in the *Guardian,* wrote that:

Art was endemic in the Lasdun family. His father, an engineer and businessman who died when Denys was only five, was a cousin of the artist Leon Bakst, who worked with the Ballets Russes. His mother was a pianist, so his childhood was spent among music and musicians.

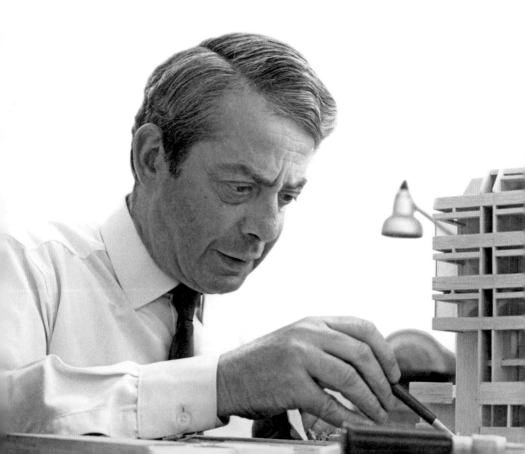

He developed what he called 'an architectural language inspired by natural geological forms'. He created forms resembling landscape formations, hills and – as he called them – 'strata'

She also described him at the Architectural Association in London, where they were both students together:

His upright carriage, the sculpted head and commanding eyes, perfectly expressed the sureness with which he was to chart his way through an embattled profession. At coffee time … Denys would not be engaged in noisy debate. He would sit with one other person, honing his architectural beliefs.

Impatient to get on with practical experience, Lasdun left the AA without completing his diploma. He worked at different times with the most significant of the architects who, in the 1930s, brought the modern movement in architecture from continental Europe to Britain: Berthold Lubetkin, Wells Coates and Maxwell Fry. At the early age of twenty-three he designed a house in Newton Road, Paddington which, drawing on Le Corbusier's Maison Cook in Boulogne-sur-Seine, was one of a small number of pioneer modernist buildings built before the war.

From the 1950s onwards he developed what he called 'an architectural language inspired by natural geological forms'. In projects like the University of East Anglia and the National Theatre, he created forms resembling landscape formations, hills and – as he called them

– 'strata'. He was profoundly inspired by ancient works, like the Greek theatre of Epidaurus, which integrate building and nature. At the same time he strongly believed that architecture should be completed by the actions of the people who used them, and saw his strata and other spaces as places to be animated by human activity.

Where earlier modernists had favoured smooth, abstract, ideally machine-made finishes, Lasdun explored rougher surfaces, such as the board-marked concrete of which the National Theatre (1967–77) is made. He also reacted against the previous generation in his attitude to the existing fabric of cities. Where the earlier attitude was often to erase and demolish, Lasdun valued the qualities in the sites where he was asked to work. His designs, while often creating strong contrasts with their settings, always respond to and engage with them.

Apart from the Royal College of Physicians, the National Theatre and the University of East Anglia, his other major works include Hallfield School, Paddington (1954), Keeling House, Bethnal Green (1960), Fitzwilliam College, Cambridge (1959–63), buildings for the University of London, and the European Investment Bank, Luxembourg (1974–80). He would say that the Royal College gave him the most pleasure of all his works.

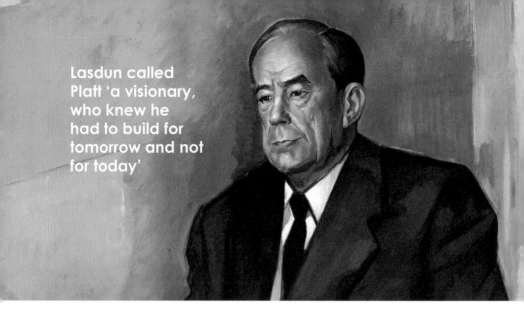

Lasdun called Platt 'a visionary, who knew he had to build for tomorrow and not for today'

ROBERT PLATT

Robert Platt (1900–78) was president of the Royal College of Physicians from 1957 to 1961 at the time that the new building project was started and Denys Lasdun was appointed architect. The completed building is a reflection of his vision of the future direction of the College and his determination and nerve in pushing the project forward.

Platt believed that the College should educate and engage with the public, for example with its report, *Smoking and Health*. This pivotal document in raising public awareness of the dangers of tobacco and in promoting policy changes, which caused a storm when it was first published, was launched at the College's first-ever press conference in 1962.

For Platt the new building should enable the College's more outward-looking culture, with its large lecture theatre and new offices. It should also symbolise change by discarding the exclusive atmosphere of its former building in favour of something more open and forward-looking. It was important to Platt, who was advised on selection by the architectural historian John Summerson, that a modern architect should be selected.

Lasdun called Platt 'a visionary, who knew he had to build for tomorrow and not for today'. For his part Platt felt the need to reassure the governing body that, although Lasdun was 'uncompromising' in his commitment to modern architecture, he would 'design a building of grace, dignity and charm that would be suitable for the College functions and traditions'.

JOHN NASH

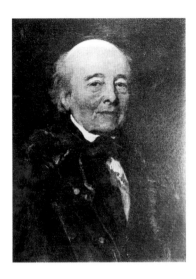

John Nash (1752–1835) was the architect who laid out Regent's Park, including fifty villas within, and the terraces fronting its edge. His work forms the setting of the Royal College: it faces the park and adjoins the predominantly Nash-designed St Andrews Place.

The park was part of a sequence of places laid out by Nash on behalf of the Prince Regent, running via Regent Street to St James's Park, which is often described as the greatest example of composed urban planning in England. It combined the classical architecture of its terraces, crescents and circuses with picturesque principles derived from garden design, particularly that of Humphrey Repton with whom Nash had collaborated for a while. As in Repton's work, Nash's planning exploits chance incidents and asymmetries, creating surprises and varied compositions.

According to John Summerson, Nash had 'a somewhat chaotic early career' as a builder/developer who was responsible for some of the first stucco-fronted houses in London. He went bankrupt, retreated to Wales and then reinvented himself as a fashionable architect of private houses and a pioneer of picturesque design. With the help of what Summerson calls 'a *mariage de convenance* which was of service to the Prince', he went on 'to fame and fortune'.

His most famous works include the Indian-style Brighton Pavilion, built as a pleasure palace for the Prince Regent, and Buckingham Palace, although the exterior visible today was rebuilt in the early twentieth century. The palace's escalating costs and Nash's complicity in the extravagance of the Prince, later George IV, caused him to fall from grace when the King died in 1830.

Nash was notoriously casual about building quality and detail and the Royal College of Physicians is more precisely and better crafted, and more solidly built, than its neighbours. But Lasdun created a rapport in his use of light and dark surfaces and in the courtyard formed by a combination of the new building and St Andrews Place. Seen from the park, as an incident within the landscape, Lasdun's building is also consistent with Nash's picturesque techniques of composition.

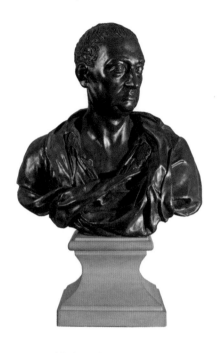

NICHOLAS HAWKSMOOR

Often cited by Lasdun as a major influence, Hawksmoor (1661–1736) was a leading figure of what was later called the English Baroque. He was a pupil of and collaborator with Christopher Wren and worked with John Vanbrugh on Castle Howard and Blenheim Palace, bringing a depth of constructional knowledge that the former playwright lacked.

He was one of the most inventive and individual British architects of all time, with a robust and uncompromising style. He combined classical with gothic elements and both with his own unique inventions. He liked to emphasise the massiveness of his buildings, and favoured abrupt changes of scale and contrasts of light and shadow.

His best-known works are the imposing churches, in bone-coloured Portland stone, that he built in east London, in particular Christ Church Spitalfields (see page 37). Nikolaus Pevsner said that this church 'cannot be called anything but ugly', but Lasdun and other post-war architects were impressed by its emotional force. On the Royal College it is possible to see the influence of Hawksmoor in its boldly projecting and recessing forms, the deep portico and use of incised lines to emphasis the surfaces.

LE CORBUSIER

Le Corbusier (1887–1965) was the most famous and influential architect of the twentieth century, whose ideas ran from the planning of cities to the design of individual buildings. He also painted, designed furniture and published and wrote extensively, promoting his ideas and works with a series of polemical texts.

In the 1920s he set out his version of what the architecture of modern times should be – it should have the precision and beauty to be found in cars, ships and aeroplanes, but also in the greatest works of ancient architecture, such as the Parthenon. It should exploit the freedoms allowed by modern construction techniques, especially reinforced concrete, and should avoid superfluous ornament and decorative motifs borrowed from the past. Architecture, he said, should enable humanity to live in fresh air and daylight, and in close contact with the natural landscape.

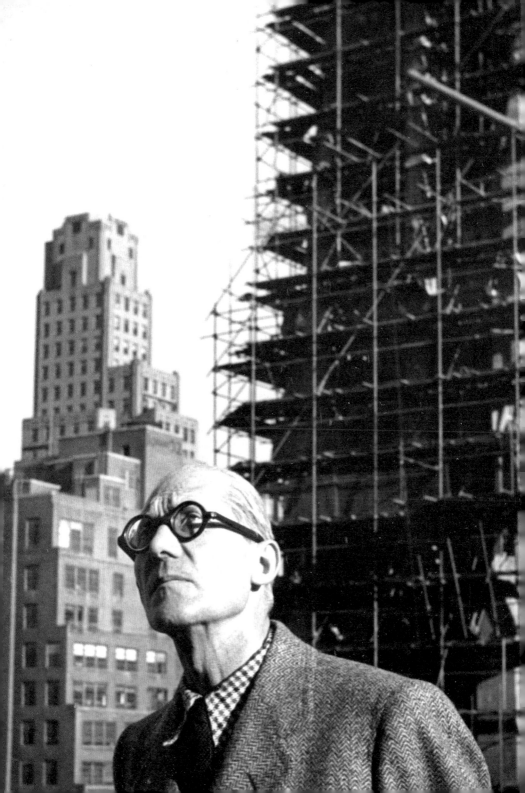

He stated these ideas in *Vers Une Architecture* of 1923, and realised them in buildings like the Villa Savoye (1929–31). He also argued for the drastic rebuilding of Paris and other cities as a series of towers and blocks set in parkland, served by high-speed roads.

Starting in the 1930s, and especially after the war, he became interested in more primitive techniques, expressive forms and rougher surfaces, while retaining his fascination with machines. The results include his government buildings for the new city of Chandigarh in India (1952–9) and the astonishing free-form church of Notre Dame du Haut in Ronchamp. He also realised a series of *Unités d'habitation*, apartment blocks which put into practice his beliefs on housing and city planning.

It became the received wisdom (now being partially revised) that he was a great creator of individual works, but that his urban theories were disastrous

As much as Le Corbusier was a hero to architects, he also became, when the reaction to modernist architecture set in, the villain. He was blamed for inhumane planning, for the actual and perceived failures of social housing built according to his theories, and for the proliferation of 'concrete monstrosities'. Even among many of his admirers, it became the received wisdom (now being partially revised) that he was a great creator of individual works, but that his urban theories were disastrous.

Lasdun, as a student at the Architectural Association, was hugely inspired by reading *Vers Une Architecture* and by a visit to Le Corbusier's Pavillon Suisse in Paris. It made him realise that 'the "dreamer"' – that is, Le Corbusier – 'could really build … it was a building that changed the course of architecture for the whole of my generation'.

He followed Le Corbusier's architecture more than his city planning, with results that can be seen in the Royal College. The aesthetic of clearly defined forms stripped of ornament is Corbusian, as is the use of reinforced concrete in construction. So is the combination of the curving, freeform Wolfson Theatre with the strictly rectangular grid of pillars supporting the main block. The strong white horizontal of the latter, elevated above the ground, has clear similarities with the Villa Savoye. There are also echoes, in the overhanging superstructure, of Le Corbusier's monastery of La Tourette, which was completed in 1959.

An architect, said Le Corbusier, 'by his arrangement of forms, realizes an order which is a pure creation of his spirit; by forms and shapes he affects our senses to an acute degree and provokes plastic emotions; by the relationships which he creates he wakes profound echoes in us, he gives us the measure of an order which we feel to be in accordance with that of our world.' This statement comes close to describing Lasdun's own philosophy.

BERTHOLD LUBETKIN

Berthold Lubetkin, born in Tblisi in 1901, arrived in London in 1931 by way of St Petersburg and Paris, where he had designed an urbane block of flats on the Avenue de Versailles. He was the most confident and talented of early modernist architects in Britain, drawing on the influences of Le Corbusier and Russian Constructivism.

Tecton, founded in 1932 and dissolved in 1948, was his practice. Its works included the Finsbury Health Centre, a pioneering project for accessible health care, and several zoo buildings, including the Penguin Pool at London Zoo. After the war they designed council housing in the boroughs of Bethnal Green, Finsbury and Paddington. In the quality of design and open space, they set standards that were rarely matched in the following decades.

It is said that Lubetkin withdrew from architecture in disgust, due to his frustrations in trying to plan Peterlee new town, and retreated to farm pigs in Gloucestershire. This is partly true, but he continued to be involved in the design of buildings until the 1960s. He died in 1990.

His influence can be felt in Lasdun's designs for the Royal College in, for example, the strong articulation and differentiation of separate elements, such as the Wolfson Theatre. The strong contrasts of light and dark, and the dynamic staircases, also owe much to Tecton.

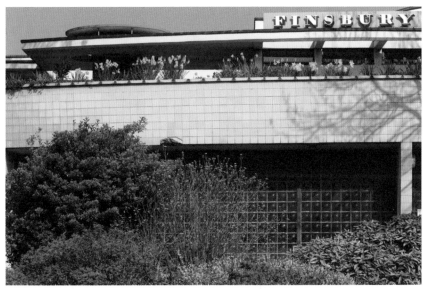

Finsbury Health Centre, London

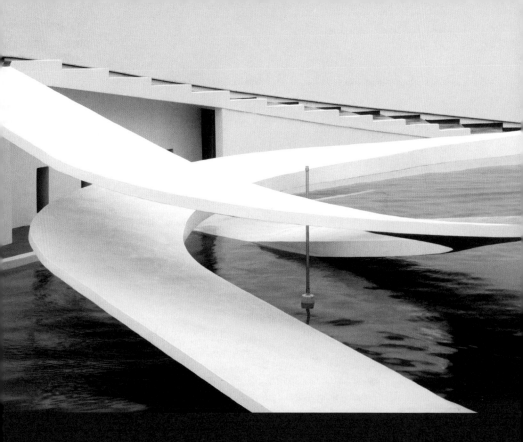

The Penguin Pool at London Zoo

OVE ARUP

Lasdun cited among his formative influences the engineers Felix Samuely, Alan Harris and, in particular, Ove Arup (1895–1988). Born in England of Danish-Norwegian parentage, and educated in Denmark, Arup played a crucial role in the development of modern architecture in Britain. Working with Lubetkin, Wells Coates and others, Arup brought the technical knowledge that made possible structures like the helical ramps on the Penguin Pool at London Zoo. At the same time he pioneered a new form of collaboration between engineers and architects in which the former would not only solve problems but also be part of the creative process.

Ove Arup founded the consultancy which bears his name and is now a vast global company, and it was the engineering practice that helped design the College. Their expertise was crucial to achieving the building's cantilevers, and it was on their advice that Lasdun was persuaded to use pillars to prop his overhanging portico. He had originally wanted that this should appear to be wholly unsupported.

PAUL KLEE

The Swiss-German artist was, as William Curtis describes, a significant influence on Lasdun at the time that the Royal College was being designed. Lasdun, writes Curtis, 'was intrigued by several of Klee's drawings and paintings around 1920 showing explosions of rectangular elements in dramatically foreshortened perspectives'. Their influence can be felt in what Curtis calls 'the hovering volumes' in the Marble Hall.

Klee (1879–1940) was an individual artist who belonged to no single school, but he was influenced by both Cubism and Expressionism. It was the Cubist qualities, of overlapping and fragmented planes, with boundaries fragmented, that most fascinated Lasdun.

THE CRITICS

The Royal College of Physicians opened to a largely positive response from both professionals and the building's users. In the *Architectural Review* the critic Robert Maxwell wrote that 'the physicians were fortunate to secure an architect who could appreciate the power and fragility of their traditions'. Lasdun, he said, 'has the rare skill of being able to create a pattern of meaningful relationships combining the psychology of use with the psychology of form', although Maxwell questioned the elaboration of its forms and doubted some of its logic. Where Lasdun argued that the brick structures such as the lecture theatre could be easily altered, Maxwell said that 'it seems as permanent as a tomb'. Of the building in general he said that 'the rationale can be betrayed by an excess of sensuous charm'.

Lasdun recorded that one Fellow 'thought the building fitted its context admirably, was generally splendid, sculpturally beautiful, but dislikes modern architecture'. The most hostile comments, in a newspaper article, were that it was a 'sausage factory' and that its elevation on Albany Street was 'a slap in the face'.

One critic with whom Lasdun had a difficult, but mutually respectful, relationship was Nikolaus Pevsner, at the time the most significant architectural writer in Britain. Pevsner, who fought for what he saw as rational architecture, thought that Lasdun and his contemporaries were introducing too much expression and emotion. Buildings like the College, said Pevsner, were 'in flat contradiction to the corpus of criteria to which … I am still committed', but he expressed his admiration for Lasdun, and recognised that the College might represent 'the legitimate style of the 1950s and 1960s'.

LOCATIONS

THE STONE HOUSE

The first home of the Royal College of Physicians was in the house of its founder Thomas Linacre, in which the College initially had the use of two rooms, as a meeting room and library. Linacre left it to the institution on his death in 1524, after which an anatomical theatre was added. The house was in Knightrider Street, south of St Paul's, and the College was based there from its foundation in 1518 to 1614.

AMEN CORNER. PATERNOSTER ROW

Amen Corner was the location of the College's second home, again in a house and also close to St Paul's, leased from the Dean and Chapter of the Cathedral. It was in use from 1614 until the building was destroyed in the Great Fire of 1666. The RCP moved there for reasons of space: it now included two rooms for anatomy lectures and accommodation for a resident fellow. In 1654 William Harvey donated his collections and money for a new library and museum. Most of the contents were destroyed in the fire, but those that survive remain in the College's possession.

WARWICK LANE

Warwick Lane was the address of the College's first purpose-built premises and was considerably larger and more architecturally ambitious than the previous two. The building was designed by Robert Hooke who, if he was overshadowed as a scientist by his enemy Isaac Newton, has been eclipsed as an architect by his friend Christopher Wren. Whereas he has sometimes been seen as a sort of technical assistant, modern scholarship tends to the view that Hooke deserves greater credit for the designs of the buildings on which he worked, including the Monument to the Great Fire.

From the surviving images the College appears to have been one of the more remarkable buildings of its time. Instead of the domestic architecture of the previous two homes, it was an orderly, symmetrical complex built around a courtyard. It had a collegiate quality and aimed to present the image of a dignified institution to the outside world – this was a place conscious of its public face, to which the public would be admitted.

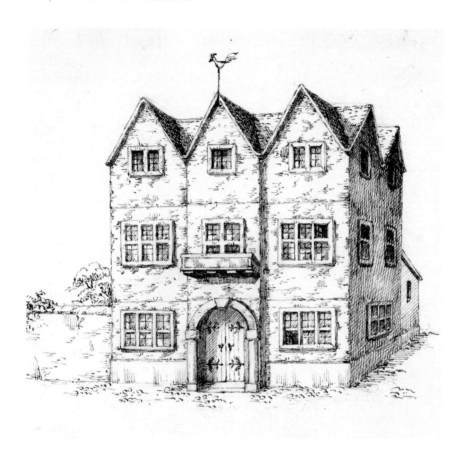

Its most striking feature was its central polygonal pavilion whose arcaded base formed the main entrance and whose superstructure contained the anatomical theatre. It is an unusual combination but also one that gives prominence to a vital part of the institution. Where the elevations of the rest of the building show an educated and competent handling of classical design, the pavilion was highly inventive – there is nothing quite like it from the period.

Built with the help of generous donations, it included the oak-panelled public gallery called the Great Room and, following the gift of the Marquis of Dorchester's collection of books in 1680, a library designed by Wren.

In use from 1675 to 1825, it was the longest lasting, so far, of the College's homes. Like the previous two it was sited close to St Paul's.

ABOVE: Amen Corner, former home of the Royal College of Physicians
FOLLOWING PAGE LEFT: The Cutlerian Theatre, Warwick Lane, former home of the Royal College of Physicians
RIGHT: Map of former Royal College of Physicians locations

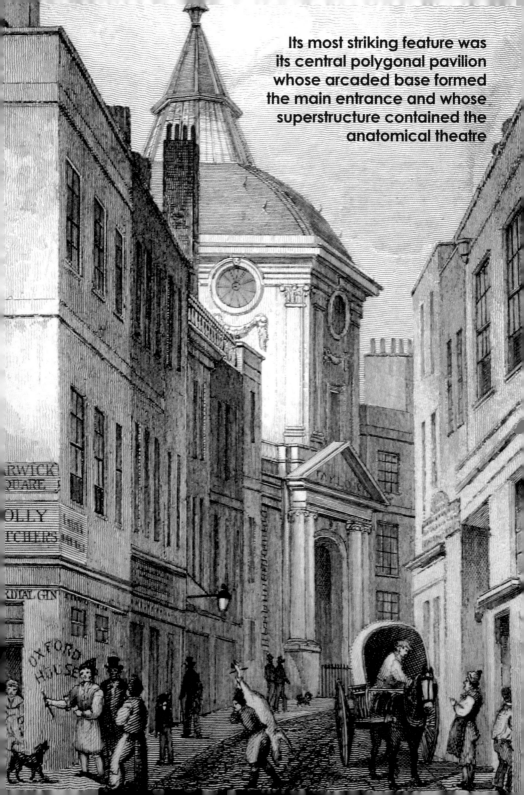

Its most striking feature was its central polygonal pavilion whose arcaded base formed the main entrance and whose superstructure contained the anatomical theatre

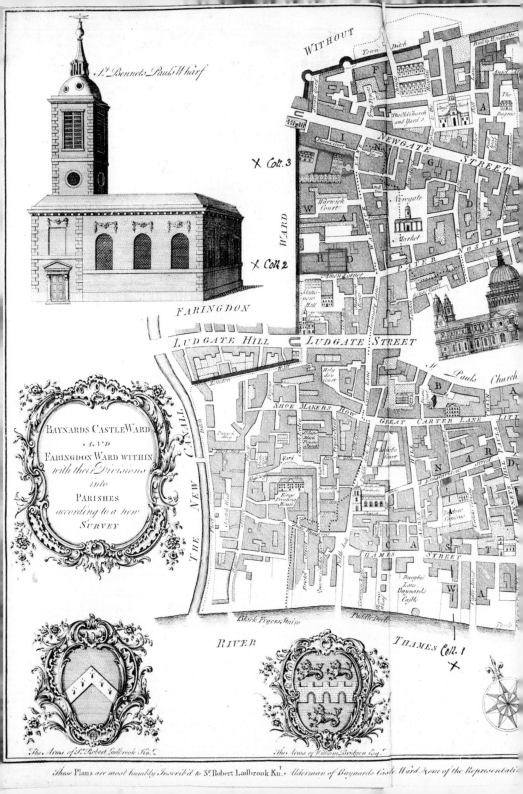

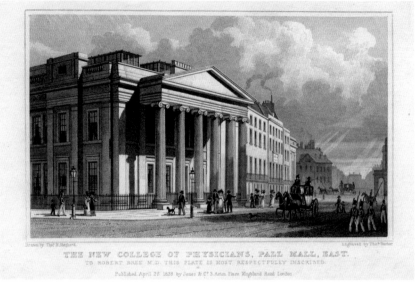

THE NEW COLLEGE OF PHYSICIANS, PALL MALL, EAST.
TO ROBERT BREE M.D. THIS PLATE IS MOST RESPECTFULLY INSCRIBED.
Published April 20 1826 by Jones & Cº 3 Acton Place Kingsland Road London

Pall Mall East, former home of the Royal College of Physicians

PALL MALL EAST

By the late eighteenth century the College's location near St Paul's had become its least attractive aspect, being unfashionable and, as John Evelyn had put it, 'obscure'. Under the president Harry Halford, who was doctor and friend to George IV, as well as treating three other monarchs, a site was found on the edge of what is now Trafalgar Square, diagonally across from the site of the future National Gallery, in an area then being re-formed by John Nash. It was a more prominent and prestigious location than any previously.

On its other side, the new building was also on the edge of what was becoming clubland and the College shared the site with the Union Club. The architect was Robert Smirke who, as well as the British Museum, designed the Carlton and Oxford and Cambridge clubs. It is therefore not surprising that, with a six-columned Ionic portico leading to a grand staircase, there should be something club-like in its character.

This was now a place for talking, meeting and studying books, rather than practical scientific work, with an impressive library and room for dining and lectures, but neither an anatomy theatre nor laboratory. In the 1920s the Canadian government took over the Union Club's part of the premises for use as its High Commission. In the 1960s they also took over the College's part of Smirke's building. It is now called Canada House.

REGENT'S PARK

Regent's Park is the culmination of John Nash's remarkable sequence of urban spaces created for the Prince Regent. For the Prince it served the interests of property speculation and aggrandisement of the monarchy, and its original plans included a royal pleasure palace and National Valhalla. John Summerson called it 'a truly remarkable conception of what we might call today a garden-city – the park landscaped on Reptonian lines, with over fifty villas half hid in groves of trees, and belted by terraces all of which had full enjoyment of the park'.

It is the primary setting of the Royal College, which was built on the site of the bomb-damaged Someries House, also by Nash. Demolition was permitted by Crown Estate Commissioners, but the new building was supposed to harmonise with its neighbours. A driving force behind Lasdun's design is its bold and dynamic engagement with his predecessor's creations.

Lasdun, however, was less impressed with the park than Summerson, at least with the view from this particular point. 'Once you've seen the view for a few minutes it's boring,' the architect said in 1960, 'there are a few trees there, it's nothing magical.' Partly for this reason the building rarely offers wide views of the park. You are aware of the greenery outside almost all the time, even from deep inside, but it is usually seen in glimpses, or filtered and layered views.

William Harvey House, 9–10 St Andrews Place

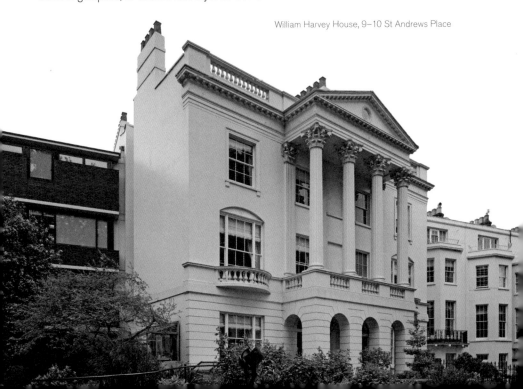

SPACES

MARBLE HALL

The heart of the College, the most complex of Lasdun's spaces there, and the one on which he devoted the most architectural energy. It is a triple height space with multiple functions: its central staircase is the main route up to places such as the Dorchester Library and the Osler Room, but it is ceremonial as well as circulatory. It is itself a social and gathering place for both formal and informal encounters. It is the place where the College represents itself: on all three levels are galleries displaying the College's collection of portraits – what Lasdun called 'the clobber of ancestral memories'.

One wall is mostly of glass, although interrupted by the cuboid containing the Censors' Room, which enables a strong connection with the exterior. It means that the Marble Hall is not a complete space in itself, but is part of a larger whole ultimately enclosed by the façade of Nash's St Andrews Place opposite. This sense is reinforced by the detail, with lines running from inside to out with minimal interruption from window frames, and the materials. The mosaic of the exterior is taken inside the Marble Hall and its Sicilian marble paving is also material you might expect to find outdoors. The hall therefore has an ambiguous, hybrid, inside/outside quality – although roofed and weatherproof it has some of the feel of a courtyard.

The palette of finishes is varied and underlines the status of the hall, and the College, with touches of luxury. As well as the marble and mosaic, there are brass handrails, doors in an east African hardwood called muninga, a ginger-coloured carpet, wall fabrics and plain plaster. The soffits of the stair and balconies were originally in white-painted cork.

From 2014, to commemorate the fiftieth anniversary of the building's completion, the Marble Hall is known as the Lasdun Hall.

The palette of finishes is varied and underlines the status of the hall, and the College, with touches of luxury

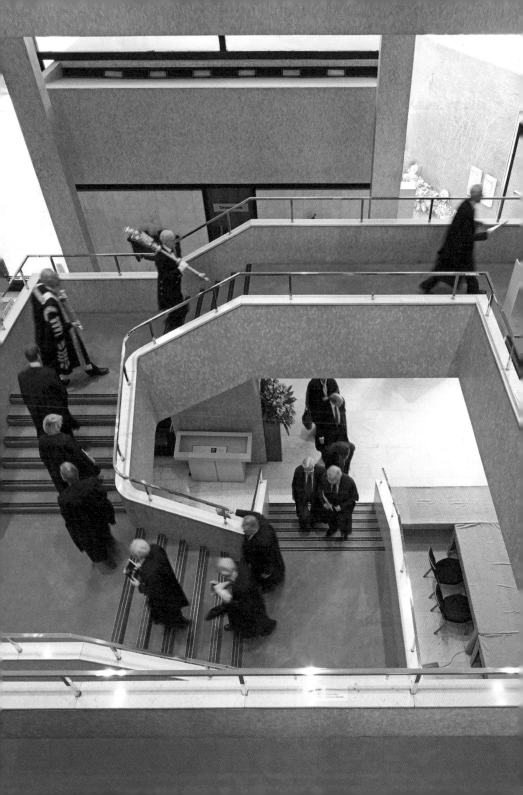

CENSORS' ROOM

From the outside, a cuboid box set within the big glass wall of the Marble Hall and projecting into the garden. Inside, a surprise, as it is lined with the Spanish oak panelling first installed in Robert Hooke's 1675 building in Warwick Lane and taken by the College as it moved to Pall Mall East and then to Regent's Park. There are also busts and gold-framed portraits by artists including Roubilliac and Lawrence, and walnut chairs donated by the president Hans Sloane (1660–1753). There is an ornate carpet and a chandelier. Somehow, despite being the antithesis of Lasdun's modern design, these traditional elements feel at home. The room is entered and exited via two small rooms, which smooth the transition, and Lasdun inserts modern vertical windows at the corner of the room, as a reminder that this is not a perfectly seventeenth-century place.

The original purposes of the Censors' Room were to conduct the demanding interview for entry to the RCP and to prosecute and discipline malpractice. These functions no longer take place there and it is now used as the starting point for ceremonial processions as well as for interviews, meetings and private lunches and dinners.

DORCHESTER LIBRARY

In 1680 the Marquis of Dorchester donated his exceptional collection of books to replace those that the College had lost in the Great Fire, on condition that a worthy space was built to house it. The first was designed by Christopher Wren, and Lasdun's version is one of the most significant spaces in the Regent's Park building. As Barnabas Calder says it is 'architecturally conservative' compared with much of the rest of the building, a symmetrical rectangular space lined with shelves set into timber panelling. It is on two levels, with a gallery running around a central double-height space. It is inward-looking and studious, lit mostly from above, with glimpses of the park allowed only through vertical slit windows at the corners.

Its most ambitious feature is not at first obvious: the upper level steps back in such a way that the lower is not overhung by the gallery. Translated to the exterior, this gives the outward-stepping form that is such a distinctive aspect of the building. To achieve this projection, and the wide unsupported span of the library's roof, was an engineering challenge, something belied by the interior's atmosphere of repose.

The library is approached on its central axis from the top of the main stair. On the wall directly opposite the entrance door is the portrait of William Harvey that was saved when the Amen Corner building burned down in 1666. The central space is kept clear for conferences, exams and other events, which can give it an empty feeling when not in use, like a disused tennis court.

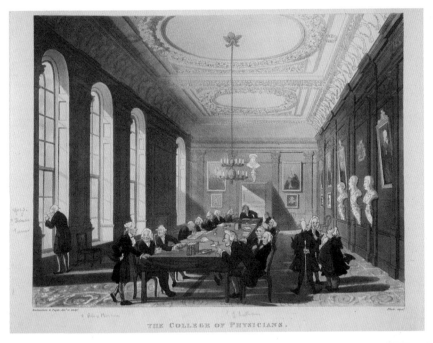

THE COLLEGE OF PHYSICIANS.

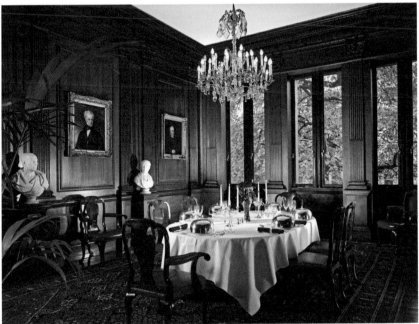

TOP: The oak panelling from the Long Room in the College's Warwick Lane home was moved to subsequent homes at Pall Mall East and St Andrews Place, where it is now in the Censors' Room (ABOVE)

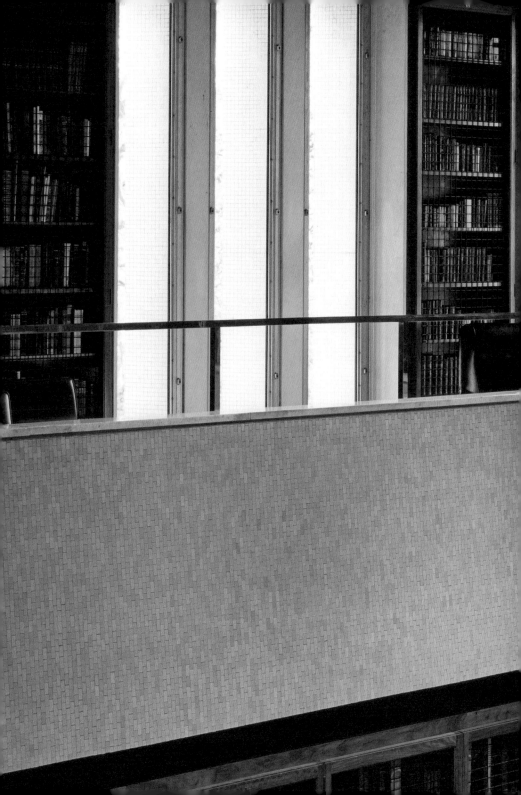

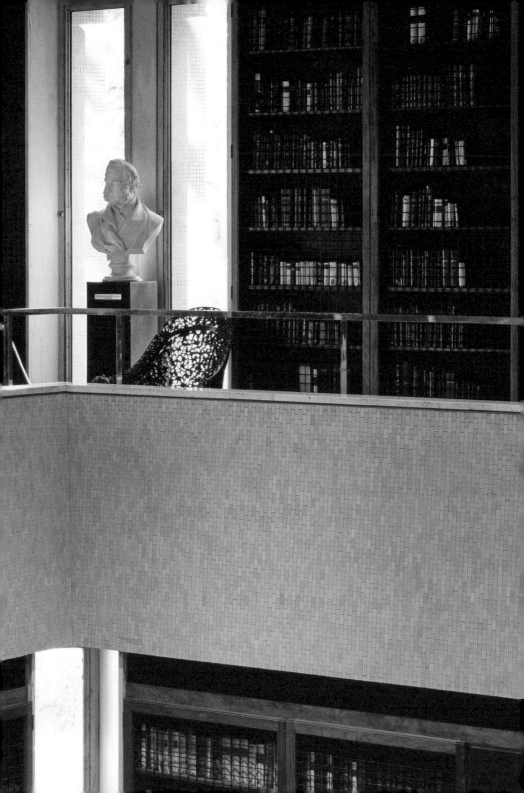

OSLER ROOM

The Osler Room is a well-proportioned double-height space with a gallery on two sides and portraits and modern art hung on the walls, which is used for banquets, exam sittings, and other functions. It is on the first floor, on the opposite side of the Marble Hall from the Dorchester Library, to which it has a roughly similar floor area. Its entrance is almost but not quite aligned with the latter's. It is reached by the main stairs, which thereby make a theatrical experience out of the ascent to dinner. Views out give glimpses of other parts of the College, in keeping with Lasdun's wish that there should be a sense of connection between different parts and that the whole building could be animated by big events.

Alongside the Osler Room is the Long Room, which is used for pre-dinner drinks and various other purposes, with generous views south over the garden. A hydraulic wall between the Osler and Long Rooms, which can rise out of the way when required, allows the two spaces to be used in conjunction.

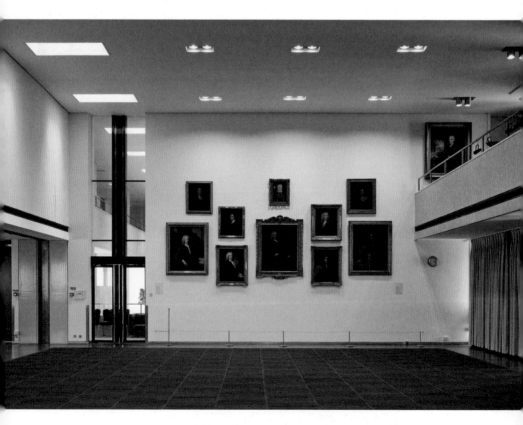

STAIRS

Each stair in the Royal College is an event and distinct from the others. There is the elegant, mosaic-clad spiral, encased in a cylinder, which leads down to the lower ground floor from the lobby of the Wolfson Theatre. There are the sequences of steps that take you gradually from ground level to the Marble Hall. There is the more functional but still spacious stair that serves the administrative offices in the rear block. There is the stair linking the first and second floors of the Marble Hall, with an intriguing hidden light source. Even the concrete escape stair attached to the north flank of the building has a sculptural dignity.

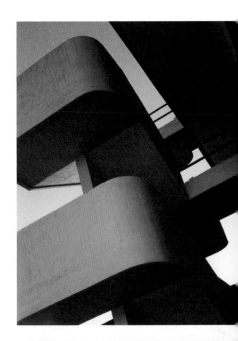

The most significant is the stair in the centre of the Marble Hall, and in the pivotal point of Lasdun's design. It is a square spiral that starts in front of the Censors' Room and ascends through three ninety-degree turns until it faces the entrance of the Dorchester Library.

Its purpose is to allow more than functional circulation: it can be a place of both chance meetings and formal ceremonies and it connects the main symbolic and social spaces of the College. As you go up, you survey the main elements of the building and comprehend its anatomy, and look out onto the Nash façade opposite. You also undertake a journey through history, with the College's ancestral portraits displayed on three of the four surrounding walls. In a delicate touch, the angles of the inner balustrade are rounded into quarter-cylinders, requiring the marble capping to be sculpted into complex forms that curve, turn and rise at the same time.

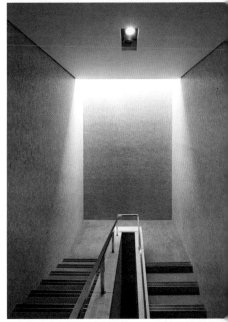

WOLFSON THEATRE

Located close to the entrance, so that the public could visit lectures without going deep into the College, the 304-seat theatre rakes downwards to a stage below ground level. Its bright white volume is unexpected, coming after a compressed, low-lit vestibule. The timber used on both the architecture and the original furnishings is Tasmanian Oak, a type of eucalyptus, donated by the Australian College of Physicians.

The theatre is wrapped in access corridors and service spaces which modify the external manifestation of its form: the sloping and curving brickwork of the exterior suggests the shape of an auditorium behind without exactly following it. In these subsidiary spaces is stored the president's throne, which Lasdun also designed.

The theatre is now used more intensively than was originally envisaged, including for conferences and events by external organisations. Its semi-detached position serves its current life well.

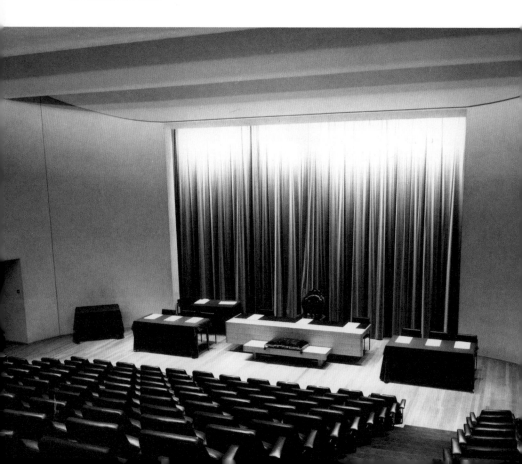

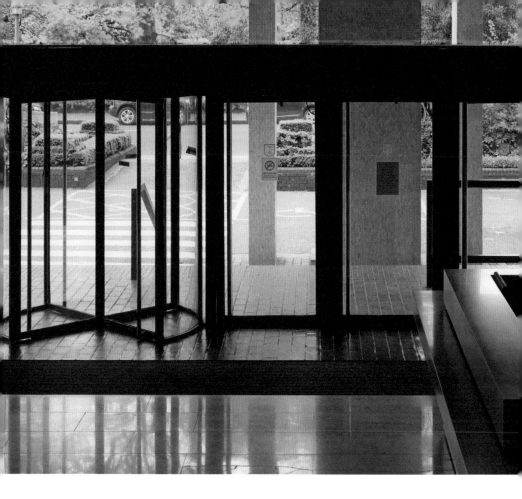

ENTRANCE HALL

A compressed and shadowy space, and deliberately so, the entrance hall contrasts with the expanses of the park, which precede it, and of the Marble Hall to which it leads. It has a hard-surfaced, half-external feel with a brick wall whose narrow penetrations give it, as several have observed, a castle-like aspect. This wall stops short of the ceiling, however, with a glass strip filling the space between, so as not to interrupt the soffit of the oversailing slab.

A right turn as you enter takes you to the Wolfson Theatre. In front you glimpse the corner of the block that contains the Censors' Room straight ahead but elevated, the beginnings of the main stair, and the first of the Marble Hall's portraits. The essential elements of the institution are hinted at, but you have to travel further to discover them fully.

OFFICE SPACE

The bulk of the offices and meeting rooms vital to the functioning of the College are concentrated in the long, relatively narrow block at the rear of the site, aligned with the terraces of Albany Street. Their design and detail is, compared to the rest of the College, unexceptional, apart from the long horizontal windows which give good views and light on both sides. Lasdun often liked to devote his architectural energies to the public parts of a building, leaving back-of-house spaces plain, which he does here.

In keeping with Lasdun's hierarchic use of materials the administrative block is expressed externally in dark brick, rather than the white mosaic used for the College's most symbolically important functions.

GARDEN

A secluded and contemplative space, reached indirectly, the garden has some of the qualities of a cloister or a College court. It has a highly specific quality, as a place for medicinal plants, that has developed since it opened in 1965. It now has over 1,300 types, from all over the world, including sixty named after doctors and apothecaries.

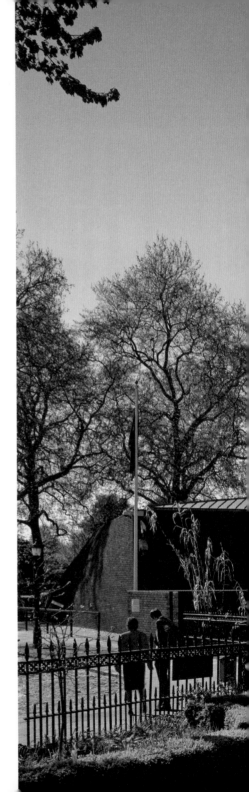

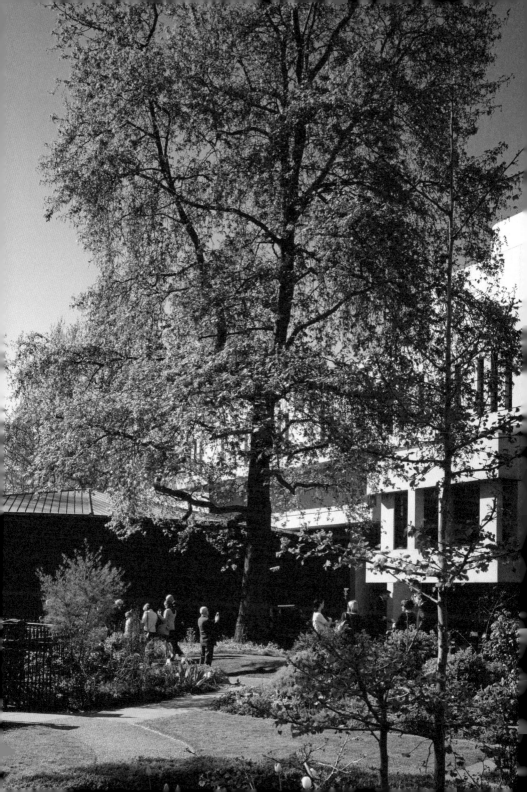

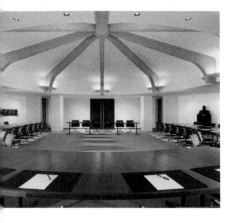

COUNCIL CHAMBER

One of Lasdun's last buildings was the addition he made to the Royal College in 1998. It is a round, domed, two-storey structure containing an additional 140-seat lecture theatre, the Seligman, below, and the Council Chamber above. Its forms and details are different from the already-diverse repertory of the original building, but it fits convincingly into the whole.

The Chamber, where the College Council meets, is sited directly opposite the Censors' Room, across the Marble Hall. It is an inward-looking space with exposed concrete ribs in its ceiling, which Lasdun compared to a monastic chapter house. Daylight comes from a concealed source, a semi-circular clerestory raised above the ceiling level, which casts its light on the wall opposite the entrance. Lasdun believed this to be one of only three 'perfect spaces' created in his career.

LOWER GROUND FLOOR

The lower ground floor contains a number of rooms, including the Buttery where staff eat every day, as do Fellows and guests when visiting. Its most significant spaces are the Seligman Theatre and the Treasures Room, a low-lit space where some of the RCP's remarkable museum collections of silver and ceremonial objects, the Symons collection of medical instruments and artefacts, and the Prujean chest – the only set of 17th century surgical instruments preserved in their original chest are on display. Just outside the room, the Victor Hoffbrand collection of apothecary jars is beautifully displayed.

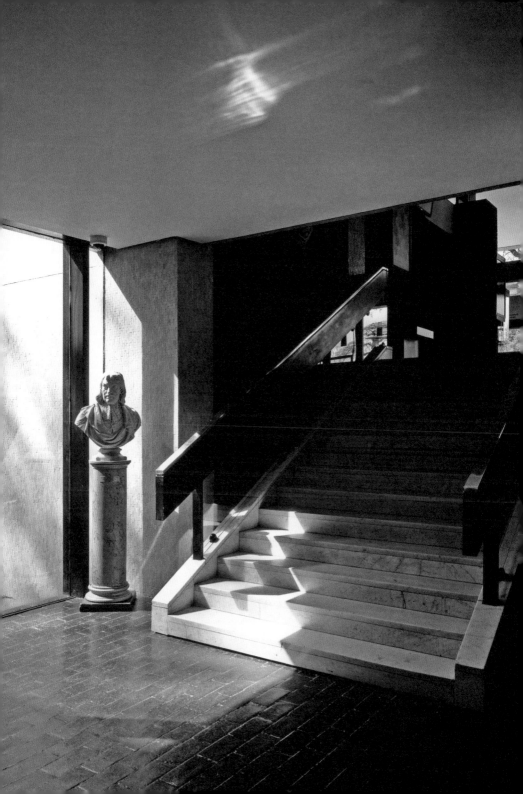

SERVICE SPACES

It is a feature of Lasdun's building that the design of cloakrooms and toilets, and their place within the whole, are carefully considered. The College was also designed at a time when mechanical services, in particular air-conditioning, were becoming increasingly significant aspects of buildings. Architects, including Lasdun, felt that these elements should be made visible, rather than suppressed. Ventilation plant and lift machinery are therefore encased in concrete and made into expressive features on the exterior.

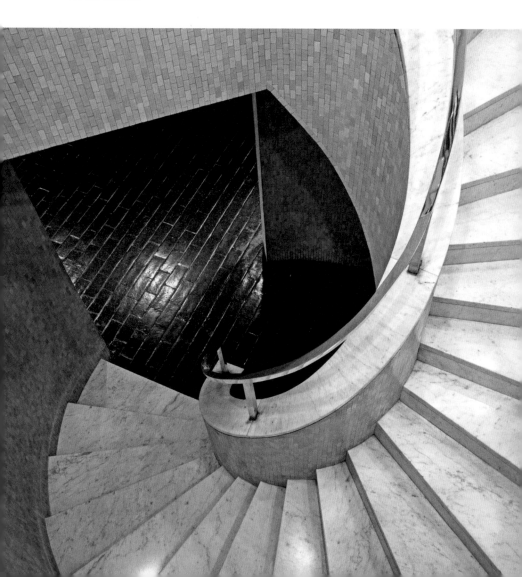

WILLIAM HARVEY HOUSE

Some of the buildings in St Andrews Place, by John Nash and George Thompson, now Grade I listed, are also occupied by the College. William Harvey House, a pedimented building at numbers 9 and 10, was refurbished in 2011 to provide eighteen bedrooms of the standard of a high quality hotel, available to fellows and staff.

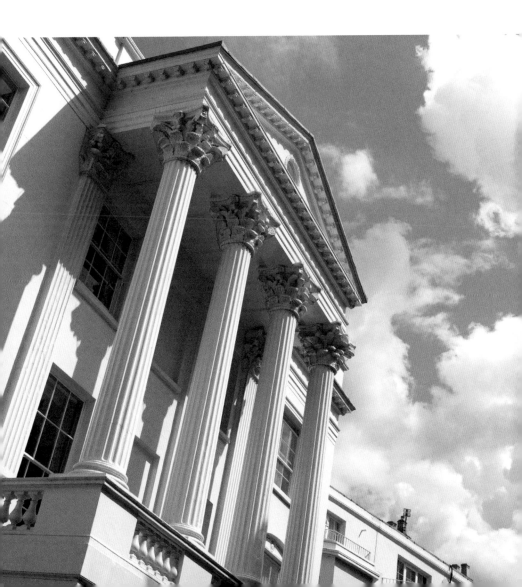

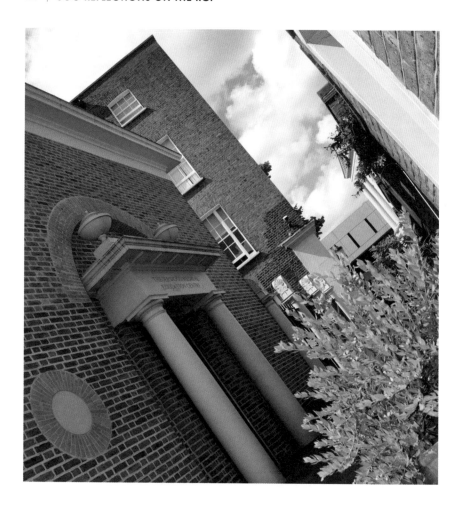

JERWOOD MEDICAL EDUCATION CENTRE

In Peto Place, just behind the College's main complex, stands the Jerwood Centre. It houses the RCP education department, which develops initiatives to improve the level of training of physicians. The building was designed by the architects Carden and Godfrey and opened in 2002. The architectural approach is very different from Lasdun's: its brick elevation, with arches and sash windows, aims to blend in with its historic surroundings.

SUBSTANCE, ELEMENTS, PROPERTIES

CLASSICISM

The classical in the design of buildings is a huge, complex and contested subject. If it might most easily be defined as the architecture of ancient Greece and Rome, or derived from these times and places, this leaves plenty of questions unanswered. In one view classicism necessarily involves the use of a particular range of ornament, including the classical orders of column. In another it embodies a philosophical belief about the relationship of humanity to the world: under this view there is more continuity between, for example, Gothic and Renaissance architecture, than stylistic details might suggest.

Another, favoured by modernists, sees classicism more as abstract principles of composition, construction and proportion, which can be realised without the use of the orders or ornament. Under this definition modern movement architects such as Le Corbusier and Mies van der Rohe saw themselves as working with classical principles. Both, for example, used variants of the trabeated form of construction used on ancient temples, composed of columns and beams made visible.

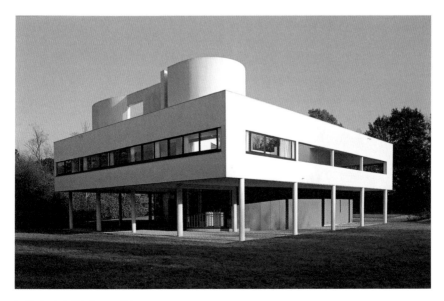

Le Corbusier's Villa Savoye, Poissy

Lasdun subscribed to this modern view. At the Royal College of Physicians the white symmetrical superstructure has some of the qualities of a classical temple. It has something resembling a trabeated structure, albeit one in which the traditional relationships of pillar to beam have greatly changed. There is however no sign of the classical orders or traditional ornament: when asked during his interview for the commission if he would include such things, Lasdun said emphatically that he would not.

THE MODERN MOVEMENT

'The modern movement' is the name given to a group of architectural tendencies which, from the early twentieth century on, sought to develop new ways of designing buildings to reflect what was seen as a time radically different from any previous – industrial, international, secular. The movement has diverse manifestations, despite attempts to codify and define it. The term can include architects highly interested in industrial construction techniques, such as the American Buckminster Fuller, or the Finn Alvar Aalto, who was more concerned with organic forms and natural building materials. It can cover functionalists, who believed that the structure and function of a building superseded all other considerations, and architects who believed in the expressive and cultural powers of design. Some architects of the modern movement were most concerned with its possibilities for reforming society, others with the design of exceptional individual buildings.

The modern movement is most commonly identified with its most famous protagonists, Le Corbusier, Mies van der Rohe and Gropius, who all combined artistic and technical ambitions. Its characteristics include the use of modern techniques such as reinforced concrete, steel frames and plate glass, the absence of ornament, flat roofs and what Le Corbusier called the *plan libre:* where traditional buildings define enclosed rooms with load-bearing masonry, modern buildings could use structural frames to create more open spaces.

The same architecture is also called 'modernist', although this label has been disliked by many of its practitioners – they believe it stresses its more superficial, stylistic qualities at the expense of its underlying concepts.

Denys Lasdun was of the second generation who, flourishing after the Second World War, both built on and questioned the ideas of the pioneers earlier in the century. The College, with its unornamented surfaces and strong forms, is clearly of the modern movement, even if it is not purely functionalist. It uses modern construction techniques, such as reinforced concrete and cantilevers, but they are not the driving force of the design as they were for some modern architects: they are used to achieve the spatial, formal and emotional qualities that Lasdun wanted to achieve.

'So far as technology is concerned,' he said, 'it is for me a repository of knowledge, an operational tool. Use it, but do not make it an end in itself.'

'So far as technology is concerned,' Lasdun said, 'it is for me a repository of knowledge, an operational tool. Use it, but do not make it an end in itself'

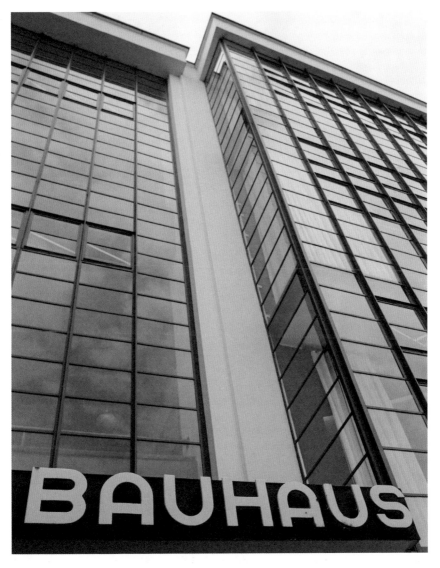

Walter Gropius's Bauhaus, Dessau

CONCRETE

Reinforced concrete became one of the defining materials of the modern movement, along with steel and glass. Originally developed for engineering and industrial purposes, its structural qualities made it appealing to architects: strong in both tension and compression, it makes possible daring cantilevers and slender supports. It also became the focus of hostility to modern architecture, attacked for its harshness and the way it stains in weather. The adjective 'concrete' became a standard prefix to the noun 'monstrosity'.

It lends itself to making strong sculptural shapes and permits a wide range of forms and treatments – it is highly responsive to architects' creative will. It was valued for being a material of modern times, as opposed to those with historical associations, such as stone. At the same time it can have an archaic or primitive quality which was increasingly appreciated as architects reacted against what they saw as the overly mechanistic or technophilic aspects of early modernism.

After the war Le Corbusier revelled in the rough surfaces concrete can have, especially when the imprint of its timber moulds is left exposed. Lasdun would also be an enthusiastic user of *beton brut*, as it is called. The College is, for him, unusually restrained in its use of exposed concrete – while the material enables the building's dramatic overhangs, much of it is covered with white mosaic. It was left visible on service elements, including mechanical plant and the escape stair, but these have now been painted to protect them from erosion.

MOSAIC

The main body of the College is clad in specially commissioned off-white porcelain mosaic, from Candolo near Turin. It creates a very different effect from the exposed concrete which, in much of Lasdun's other work, would be the principal external finish. Where concrete weathers, mosaic remains largely unchanged and it has the effect of lightening the apparent mass. It brings a refinement that reflects both the dignity of the institution and the sensitive location next to Nash's terraces.

It is used to define the more elevated functions of the College, such as the Dorchester Library and the Marble Hall, and is put into strong and deliberate contrast with the dark, rough-surfaced brickwork of the lower and rear parts of the building.

The mosaic goes against the architectural preferences of the time, which were for the raw and the rough. Robert Maxwell, in the *Architectural Review,* wasn't sure about it: it has 'a lightness and a slickness which are painterly rather than sculptural', he said, and also called it 'a flimsy covering, an outer garment of druidic linen'.

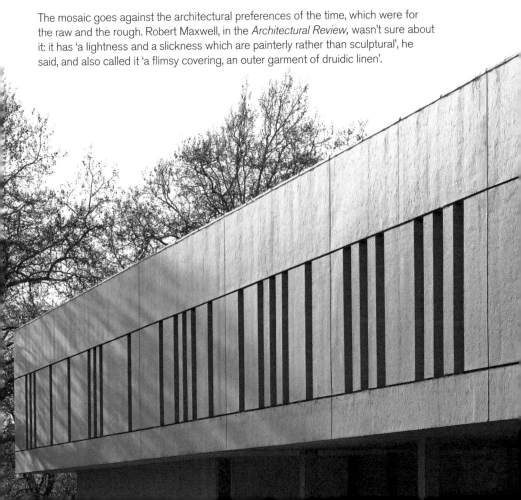

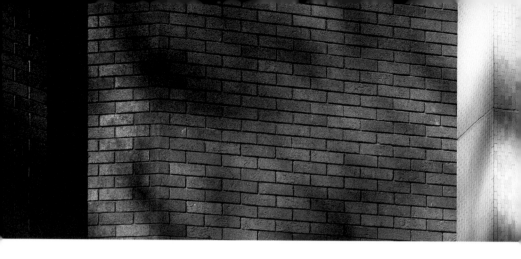

BRICK

Brick is one of the most traditional, not to say ancient, materials, its essential character unchanged for millennia. A brick's approximate dimensions vary little over time – if bigger it would be too big for builders to handle it easily; if smaller it would require more joints and be more laborious to assemble.

It is one of the principal materials of the College, used for lower levels, those closer to the outside world, and for the administrative parts of the building. It is also used for paving and for planters. Lasdun closely associates it with the earth and the ground, and strongly contrasts it with the white mosaic that clads the most elevated functions of the building. Its rough, tactile surface, which you experience on first approaching the College, also contrasts with the more refined finishes inside.

The extensive use of brick can be seen as an example of post-war architects' reaction against the smooth, mechanical aesthetic of earlier modernism. That chosen by Lasdun is, however, blue-black engineering brick from the Baggeridge works in Staffordshire, whose hardness and strength makes it suitable for railway and factory building. It therefore has the feel of engineering, unlike the mellow yellowish-brown stock brick of which much of London is built.

Lasdun then uses it with precision and refinement, demanding high levels of skill from its layers. Thirty-seven different types of brick, individually designed and specified, were needed on the building, including those used to achieve the complex shape of the wall of the Wolfson Theatre. Lasdun also uses this hard material counter-intuitively to make the curving, soft-looking forms of the theatre's wall, whereas the mosaic-clad concrete structures are mostly rectilinear. As bricks are oblong and most easily laid in vertical walls, and concrete is mouldable, you might expect the roles to be reversed.

ART

As well as being a medical organisation, the Royal College of Physicians holds a significant collection of over 5000 works of art, in particular portraits of presidents and fellows, and others associated with the College. The display of at least some of these works was an important consideration in the design of the building and they play a prominent role in the architectural experience of the interior.

The College also has works of post-war art, including the large abstract by John Hoyland that hangs in the Osler Room, and the heraldic stained glass window that you encounter on the right as you approach the Marble Hall. This is by Keith New (1925–2012) who, as a recent graduate from the Royal College of Art, was commissioned with two others to create the stained glass windows for the nave of the new cathedral at Coventry. His commission for the Royal College of Physicians was more modest but its bright multicoloured light, in which blue, red and yellow dominate, create a striking and unexpected moment in Lasdun's architecture. It is characteristic of the building's design, which is emphatic but not over-controlling, that it happily accommodates both New's glass and fragments from the RCP's former homes that can be seen on the first floor gallery.

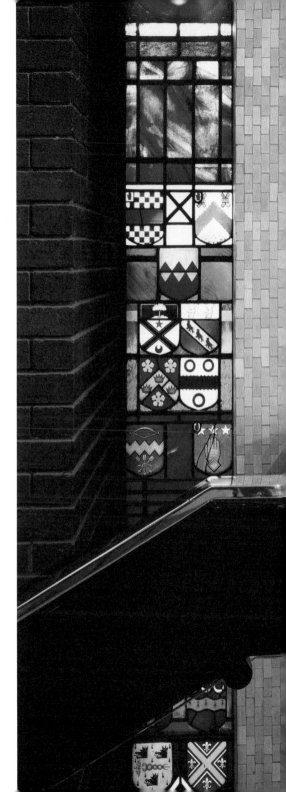

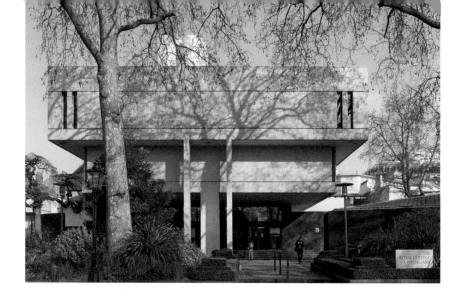

FRONT

William Curtis sees in the front of the College the influence of the East End churches of Nicholas Hawksmoor. Like their entrance elevations, it offers both flatness and depth, with almost-blank expanses of off-white undercut by a deep, shadowy portico. It is forbidding and welcoming at the same time and makes sure that you know that you are entering an exceptional place. The first flight of steps, leading to a wide platform on which you can pause before entering, starts a slow ascent that will continue inside.

The balance of verticals and horizontals is completely different from Hawksmoor's, but both architects liked to create a forceful interplay between the two. Like the churches, the College offers a dramatic profile to the approaching visitor.

The portico of the College likes to confound expectations. It looks axial and symmetrical except that, at the central point where a classical building would make the entrance, there is a bunching of three pillars and the front door is offset. The design is frontal, suggesting that it should be addressed head-on, but the main approach is oblique, the better to appreciate the shapes it makes against the sky.

In this tangential approach to a symmetrical structure, which is also part of a group of objects, it is not too fanciful to see the influence of the Acropolis, as described in *Vers Une Architecture*. There Le Corbusier shows how the Parthenon, with smaller temples around it, can be seen but not reached directly – the experience of the place unfolds by moving through it. Lasdun then creates another version of the suggestive group of volumes, which require further exploration, on entry into the building, where you can see part but not all of the Censors' Room and other crucial elements.

BACK

The rear block of the College, on Albany Street, is one of its most controversial aspects. It replaced ten Georgian houses with administrative offices rendered externally with strong alternating bands of glass and engineering brick. It contrasts strongly with its vertically proportioned, light stucco neighbours in a way that was criticised by Basil Spence, architect of Coventry Cathedral, when the design was assessed by the Royal Fine Arts Commission, the public body that then advised on significant architectural projects. Lasdun was unmoved.

This elevation is hard to justify according to many rules of townscape and conservation, but is handsome in itself, and makes sense as part of the larger ensemble of College structures. It announces a shift from domestic buildings to institutional and plays a part in the interplay of the new and old buildings, which proceeds by a combination of likenesses, contrasts and inversions.

The blunt backside was a recurring feature of Lasdun's buildings: the National Theatre and his Christ's College buildings both had cliff-like rears, both now to varying degrees obscured by later structures.

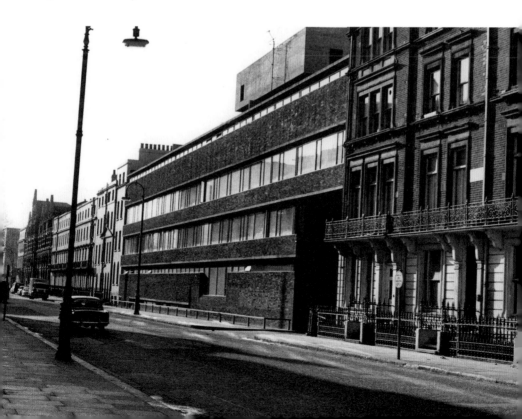

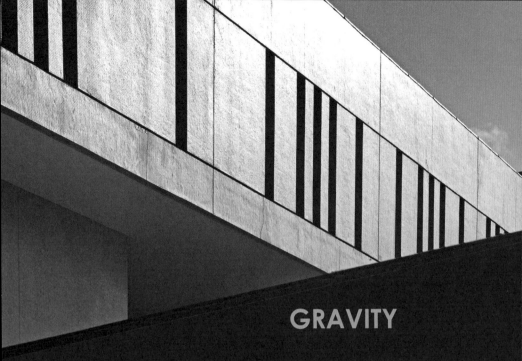

GRAVITY

The denial and acknowledgement of the demands of gravity is a theme running through Lasdun's design, exploited to give emotional and expressive range. He uses cantilevers to make large masses hang, seemingly impossibly, in the air. He had hoped to achieve the deep overhang at the entrance entirely without vertical supports, eventually settling for a group of three uprights that still look too spindly for their task.

He also used a grid of slender pillars, similar to Le Corbusier's use of cylindrical *pilotis*, to support the building. In the Marble Hall these become visible and significant elements, used to define and give order to the space. The mound-like shape of the Wolfson Theatre seems to emphasise its earthbound weight.

The effect is to heighten awareness of the forces at play in the structure, sometimes to unsettle and sometimes to affirm expectations.

ENTABLATURE

In classical architecture, the entablature is the horizontal element placed above columns. It is integral to the five orders of architecture, with specific ornamental details associated with each. Thus the Doric includes triglyphs in its entablature – the vertical, three-grooved tablets underpinned by peg-like *guttae*, which recall the beam-ends of timber construction.

The horizontal superstructure of the Royal College has memories of a classical entablature, though its proportions in relation to the slender uprights that support it are greatly distorted. It is possible to see echoes of triglyphs in the spacing of vertical windows.

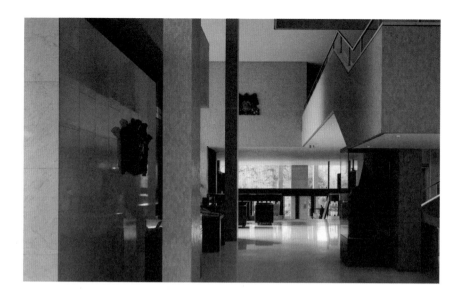

PROMENADE ARCHITECTURALE

The *promenade architecturale* is the idea, with origins in landscape architecture, and developed by Le Corbusier, that a building should not be experienced from a single viewpoint but should be revealed by movement through it. The Royal College of Physicians is a complex and sophisticated realisation of this idea, with a series of contrasts of spaces that are expansive or compressed, open or closed, high or low, and dark or light, and which offer different relationships to the surroundings. It can only be comprehended through several journeys in and around the building.

TRANSPARENCY AND OPACITY

The College's ambitions for the building included the desire to make it more open and accessible to the public, in contrast with the exclusive aspect of Smirke's building in Pall Mall East. Transparency was a powerful idea from early in the modern movement and in recent decades it is common for architects to interpret such a brief with the extensive use of glass to show the inner workings of the organisation. Lasdun uses transparency more selectively. He first presents an exterior with surprisingly few windows, which the critic Robert Maxwell described as 'opaque'. As you get to the building, however, and then as you pass inside, it opens up. It is accessible, but it doesn't want to reveal everything at once. It enforces the idea that this is a special place for an exceptional institution, not to be entered thoughtlessly.

INSIDE/OUTSIDE

A favourite device of twentieth-century architects is the flow of space from inside to out, the overlapping of the two and the blurring of distinctions between them. Frank Lloyd Wright and Mies van der Rohe, for example, would both pursue these effects, through using glass walls, external materials indoors and strong horizontals, with frames and other details minimised at the point of transition. Lasdun, who on his honeymoon in Chicago both toured the work of Wright and met Mies, employed all these methods on the College.

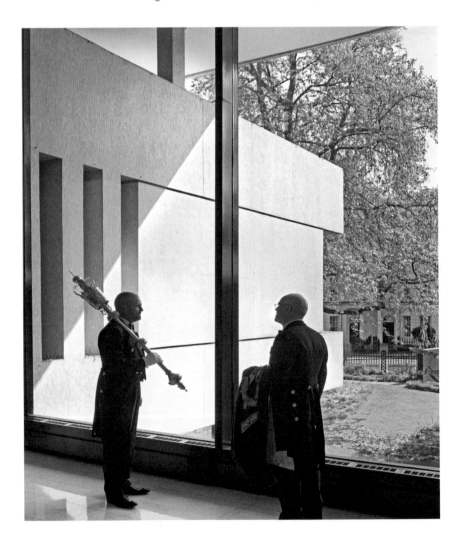

PLAN

One of the three types of drawing, the others being section and elevation, with which the organisation and form of buildings is usually described. The plan, which might be said to set out the anatomy of a building, had a particular importance for modern movement architects as being the means by which the architectural concept is established. 'The plan is the generator, and proceeds from in to out,' said Le Corbusier, by which he meant that the external appearance of the building should be a consequence of its internal structure.

The College follows these principles: its plans clearly express the various elements of the building while ordering them within an overall structural rhythm. Even without close study, it is possible get from them a sense of the building's hierarchy.

SECTION

Lasdun, along with other architects of his generation, also placed importance on the cross-section. The cross-section of the College is rich and varied, with volumes of different heights, reflecting their use and status, several changes of level and variable roof heights on the exterior. The relationships between these volumes and levels, their interlocking and their contrasts, does much to shape the experience of the building. There is, for example, the gradual ascent as you enter the building from the ground level up two flights into the Marble Hall, where the space is first compressed, then opens up into the triple-height volume of the hall.

ELEVATION

The least important of the three types of drawing, according to modernist principles. It was particularly taboo to design from the outside in – to consider first the external effect of an elevation or façade and then try to make the internal functions fit. In keeping with these ideas, Lasdun's elevations follow from and articulate the plan and section. They are, however, highly considered and composed and the effects of critical details, such as the incised lines in the mosaic surface, are precisely judged. Even where the plan is given priority, architectural design in fact involves working in all directions between plan, section and elevation, to explore how each affects the other.

First floor

Second floor

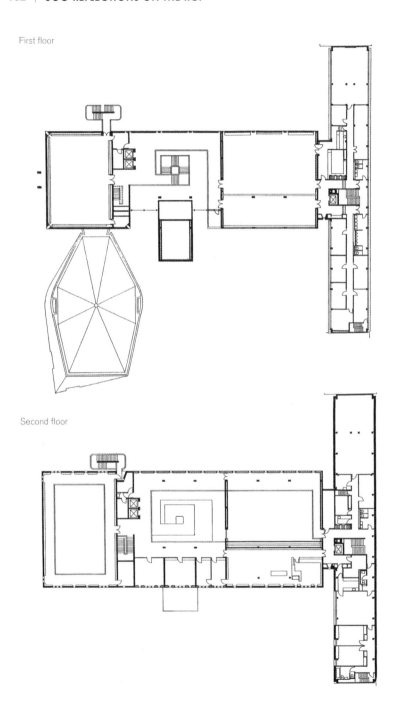

Longitudinal

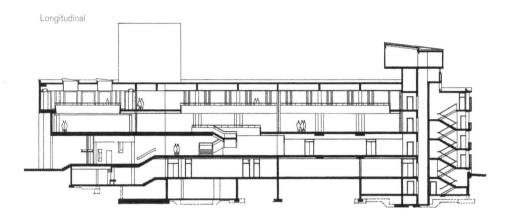

Architectural design involves working in all directions between plan, section and elevation, to explore how each affects the other

Traversal

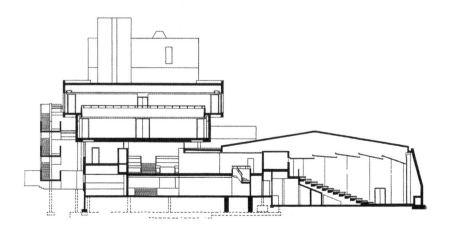

THE HORIZONTAL

The College's emphasis is strongly horizontal, both inside and out. A series of planes or layers are established with devices such as the overhanging portico, the balconies in the Marble Hall and the long windows on Albany Street. At the same time the visitor's progression through the building usually takes the form of a more or less gradual ascent. There are also the plunges down, not always expected, of the spiral stair next to the Wolfson Theatre, and of the seating in the theatre itself. What looks from the front like a three-storey building turns out to have, in places, five.

The effect is to heighten awareness of upward or downward movement and give significance to the act of passing deeper into the institution. Circulation is not treated as a purely functional or thoughtless act, but is given meaning. At the same time the College's horizontals anticipate Lasdun's later development, especially on the National Theatre, of the idea of 'strata': layers inspired by geology, forcefully expressed, which are the settings of human activity.

LIGHT

The effects of light are crucial to the experience of the College building and, as with other aspects, Lasdun works with extremes and their reconciliation. A powerful contrast of light and dark is established with the brick and mosaic of the exterior, which is then restated by the progression from the shadowy entrance into the bright Marble Hall.

Light has several properties and manifestations in the building. There is the inundation of sunlight, casting strong shadows, through the south-facing glass wall of the Marble Hall and the more muted top-light of the Dorchester Library, augmented by narrow vertical windows. The Council Chamber, with its concealed overhead light source, offers something else again. At night, if the Marble Hall is illuminated within, the masses of the building seem in the external view to dematerialise.

In sunlight the overhanging external forms cast strong and defined shadows, while trees throw lighter and more mobile patterns on the mosaic planes. 'Architecture', said Le Corbusier at the outset of *Vers Une Architecture*, 'is the masterly, correct and magnificent play of masses brought together in light.' Lasdun would not have forgotten this statement when designing the College.

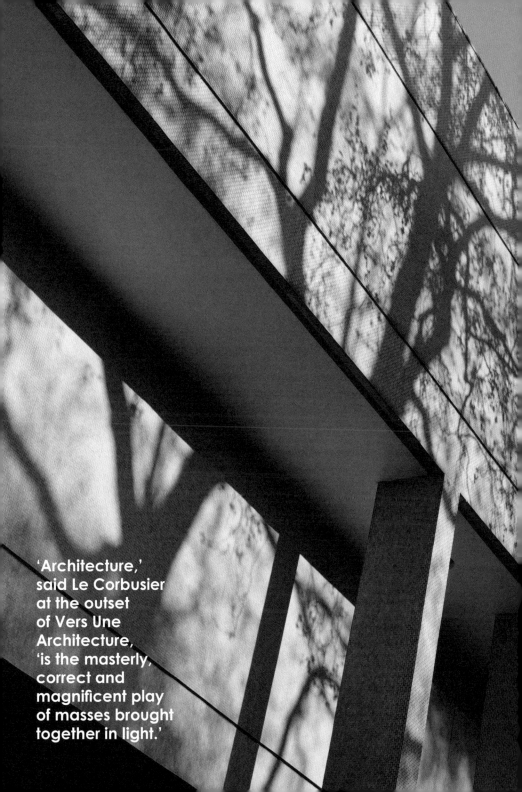

'Architecture,' said Le Corbusier at the outset of Vers Une Architecture, 'is the masterly, correct and magnificent play of masses brought together in light.'

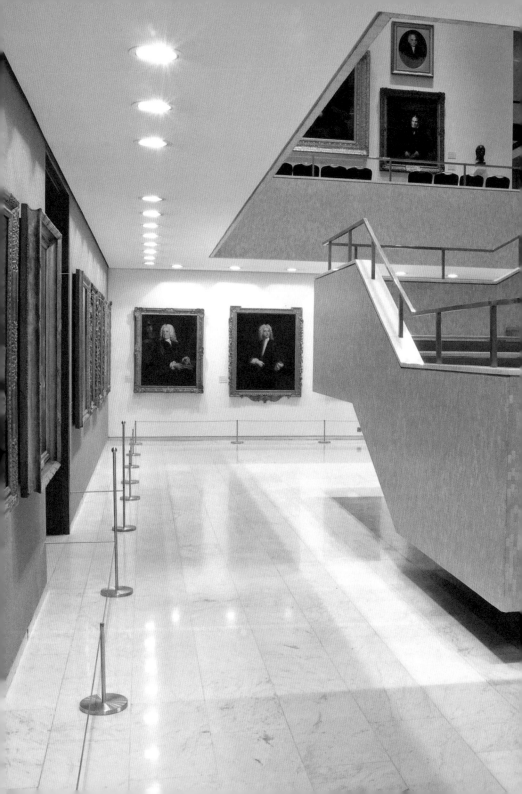

SCALE

A sense of scale is far from lacking in Lasdun's design, but it can be inscrutable. There are not the clues given by traditional ornament or conventional windows and doors and the first reading is ambiguous: it looks like a three-storey building – that is, something not very big – but the storey heights are large ones. The slit windows, in their unfamiliarity, are hard to decipher. You might guess that they are about the height of a man, but you'd be wrong. They are bigger.

At the same time the descent in scales, from that of the building to that of the entrance, is scrupulously, almost musically modulated, through a series of similarly proportioned but reducing rectangles. The top face of the portico is larger than the one below, which is larger than the framing in which the doors are set. Other rectangles, and the lines incised in the surface, supplement these relationships.

There is also an inconspicuous building-up of masses. As you first walk off the pavement into the territory of the College, planters join you on the left, knee-high or less, built of the same brick which grows on the right-hand side into the curving brick wall of the theatre, which is of a scale with, but subordinate to, the white blocks of the main structure. It guides you into the entrance, from where there is a further ascension and declension of volumes. The patterns of bricks and mosaic add further registers of scale.

LUXURY

Some of Lasdun's buildings, including his council housing and the new University of East Anglia, were built to limited budgets. The Royal College answers to its members rather than the taxpayer and so, without being irresponsible, felt the need for finishes equal to its dignity. As a result luxurious elements are employed to an extent rare both in Lasdun's other work and in most architecture of the 1960s: marble, mosaic, brass, bronze and the different kinds of hardwood, from Britain, Africa and Australia.

In addition to the quality of the materials there is the crafting. Lasdun's design makes demands of its makers, in its precision throughout, in the elegant spiral stair that descends from the lobby of the Wolfson Theatre, in the three-dimensional shaping of the marble capping to the balustrade of the main stair, in its ambitious cantilevers and in the leaning, curving brickwork of the exterior.

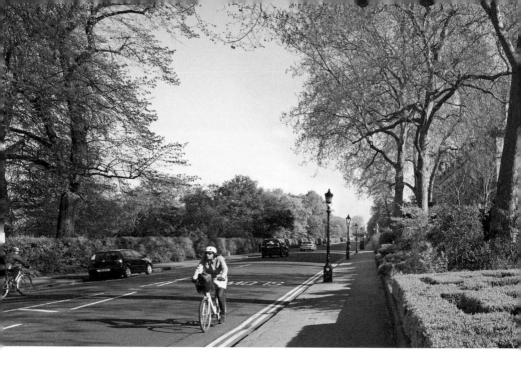

THE ONE-OFF

A recurring idea of twentieth-century architecture, which continues into the present, was the idea of the repeatable design. It was hoped that techniques of mass production could create better, cheaper buildings more efficiently than before, just as industrial processes had done with the manufacture of cars. The idea was popular when Lasdun's career was at its peak, and he was sensitive to criticism on this point – in 1965 he observed that 'one-off' had 'come to be a dirty word'.

In many projects, including the University of East Anglia and his building for Christ's College, Cambridge, he experimented with repeatable elements, but he was above all concerned with designing specific buildings in particular places for specific users and clients. His building in Regent's Park is an outstanding example of this: a mass-produced Royal College of Physicians, a building type that is required on average once per century, would be nonsensical. His design was bespoke, highly tailored both to the requirements of the brief and to the location.

Allied to the enthusiasm for mass-produced construction was a social concern – the belief that it was better to create repeatable designs that could serve as many people as possible, rather than singular 'prestige' projects. Lasdun argued that all buildings, however modest, deserved the same respect and that 'the lifeblood of the exchange of information with the building user' was, for him, 'sacred'. He welcomed more efficient techniques, but believed that they should serve, not replace, this relationship.

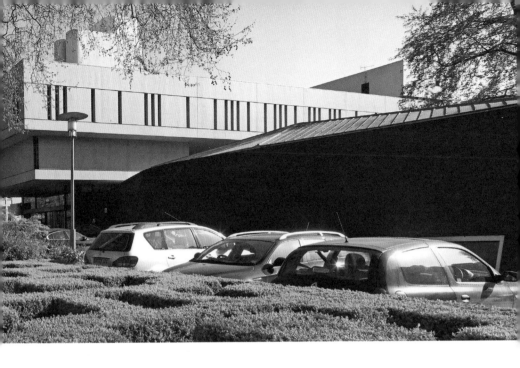

PERMANENCE AND CHANGE

In the composition of the College, Lasdun distinguished between those elements that he saw as fixed and those that might be changed over time. The first was defined by the rectangular, symmetrical and elevated structure clad in white mosaic, which has what one critic called 'the finality and the dignity of completed and unchanging essences'. The second is expressed by the free-form, asymmetrical, lower structures in dark brick. He also used exposed concrete (now painted) to denote ventilation structures, the escape staircase and other service elements.

In this he reflects what was then an emerging concern for the adaptability of buildings and the increasing role of mechanical services, which would be more fully expressed in the Pompidou Centre over a decade later. On the College (as indeed on the Pompidou Centre), the differentiation is symbolic more than practical. As critics have pointed out, the massive and hard-to-build structure of the Wolfson Theatre would not be lightly altered. Lasdun's concept was, however, vindicated by the addition in the 1990s of the Council Chamber and the Seligman Theatre: a substantial new structure that was added without damaging the original building's architectural intent.

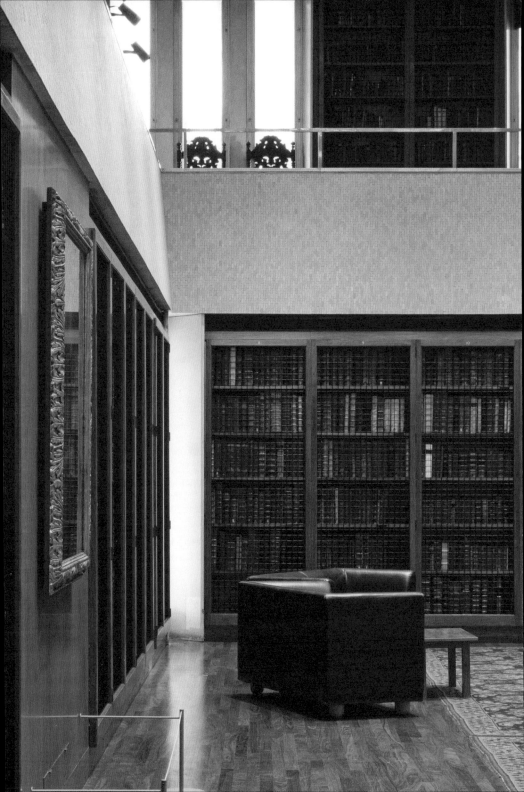

BIBLIOGRAPHY

This book is particularly indebted to Barnabas Calder's knowledgeable and perceptive book on the Royal College of Physicians building, *A Monumental Act of Faith*. It aims to build on and interpret Calder's discoveries rather than repeat them.

A language and a theme: the architecture of Denys Lasdun & partners. London: RIBA Publications, 1976.

Banham, R., *The New Brutalism*, Architectural Review, December 1955

Briggs A. *A history of the Royal College of Physicians of London: volume four*. Oxford: OUP, 2005.

Calder B. *Denys Lasdun's Royal College of Physicians: a monumental act of faith*. (edited by Emma Shepley) London: Royal College of Physicians, 2008.

Curtis WJR. *Denys Lasdun: architecture, city, landscape*. London: Phaidon Press, 1994.

Harris, S., *Nikolaus Pevsner: the Life*, Pimlico, 2013

Lasdun D. An architect's approach to architecture. *RIBA Journal* 1965;72:184-95.

Lasdun D. Architecture, continuity and change. *RIBA Transactions* 1982:27-35.

Lasdun D. Completing the College. *Journal of the Royal College of Physicians of London* 1996;30:293-5.

Le Corbusier, *Toward an Architecture*, Getty Publications 2007

Maxwell R. Royal College of Physicians, Regent's Park, London . *Architectural Review* 1965;137:268-80

Medical mores: Royal College of Physicians extension, Regent's Park, London. *Architectural Review* 1997;202:77-9.

Rowntree, D., *Obituary: Sir Denys Lasdun*, The Guardian, 12th January 2001.

Scott, G., *The Architecture of Humanism*, W.W.Norton, 1914.

Summerson, Sir John, *Architecture in Britain, 1530 to 1830*. London: Penguin Books, 1954

Webb M. Royal College of Physicians. *Country Life*, 1964.

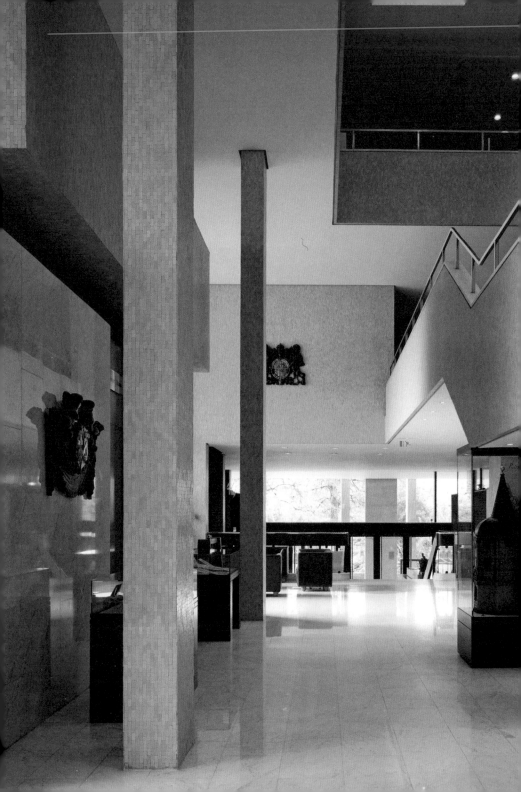